WITHDRAWN

Outsourcing
in Health Care

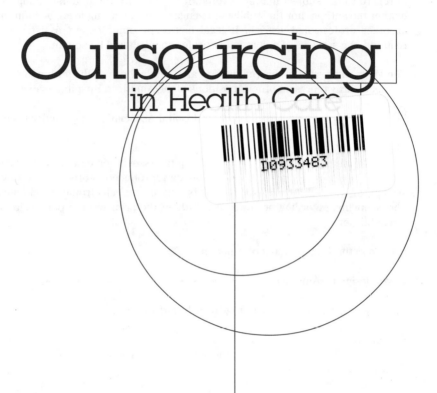

The
Administrator's
Guide

Jo Surpin and
Geri Weideman

press

Health Forum, Inc.
An American Hospital Association Company
Chicago

This publication is designed to provide accurate and authoritative information in regard to the subject matter covered. It is sold with the understanding that neither the authors nor the publisher is engaged in rendering legal, accounting, or other professional service. If legal advice or other expert assistance is required, the services of a competent professional should be sought.

The views expressed in this publication are strictly those of the authors and do not necessarily represent official positions of the American Hospital Association.

Printed in the United States of America—1/99

Cover design by Amy Aves

Library of Congress Cataloging-in-Publication Data

Surpin, Jo.
    Outsourcing in health care : the administrator's guide / by Jo
Surpin and Geri Weideman.
        p.   cm.
    Includes index.
    ISBN 1-55648-251-5 (pbk.)
    1. Hospital care—Contracting out.   I. Weideman, Geri.
II. Title.
RA971.3.S87   1999
362.1'068'1—dc21
DNLM/DLC
for Library of Congress   98-47917
                                                                        CIP

Item Number: 162300

Contents

About the Authors

Jo Surpin is president of MEDIQ Consulting Group, Pennsauken, New Jersey. She has directed strategic planning initiatives, including the creation of multihospital systems, service reconfiguration, and development of implementation plans. In addition to the hospital setting, she has been involved in projects involving ambulatory care centers, physician practices, and managed care organizations. In each of these settings, she has assisted health care providers in using outsourcing as a mechanism to improve the efficiency and effectiveness of operations. MEDIQ also provides outsourcing services by offering management services to ambulatory care facilities and freestanding imaging centers. Ms. Surpin has also been involved in developing and implementing business plans for other MEDIQ companies, including asset management services and biomedical engineering.

Ms. Surpin has lectured and written extensively on planning and reimbursement issues and published numerous articles on strategic planning initiatives, managed care strategies, and new service development for hospitals. She has lectured for various local and national professional associations/societies and universities. She has coordinated large-scale training and technical assistance programs and has conducted numerous retreats for hospital boards and regional planning agencies. Ms. Surpin has coauthored a book on diagnosis-related group rate setting for New Jersey hospitals and founded the *DRG Monitor*, a national newsletter on prospective payment issues. Ms. Surpin holds a master's degree in economics from Temple University in Philadelphia. She is a board member for a number of organizations, including the Pennsylvania College of Optometry and MRI of San Luis Obispo, California.

Geri Weideman is a senior consultant with MEDIQ Consulting Group, involved in operations assessment, activity projections, and management redesign, including analysis of work flow, staffing, and cost reduction. She has been actively involved in the research and design of databases to provide benchmark information for a variety of hospital departments. She coordinates the firm's consulting activities in performing operational audits for multihospital systems' asset management and logistics programs. She has been involved with other MEDIQ companies, assisting in the development of business plans for opportunities in asset management and biomedical engineering. She is also involved in providing research services.

Ms. Weideman has written and lectured on a variety of topics, including outsourcing and group purchasing organizations. Prior to her work with MEDIQ, she was a consultant in nonsalary cost reduction. She also has served as materials manager and nurse manager in an urban teaching facility.

Ms. Weideman holds a diploma in nursing from Albert Einstein Medical Center in Philadelphia, a BS in health management from Saint Joseph's University, and a masters of business administration from Temple University. She is a member of the American Society of Health Care Materials Managers.

Preface

Outsourcing is a strategy that can be used to respond to the challenges that must be dealt with in the current health care environment. Health care administrators and managers must be familiar with methodologies and procedures that will help them to deal with the changing world in which they operate. From middle managers to the chairperson of the board, health care executives must be prepared to quickly change direction, respond to change, and move forward. Outsourcing can be a tactic to achieve the goals of the institution while reducing costs.

Outsourcing is not a new management tactic, although its application in certain areas of health care is relatively new. Corporations in a variety of industries have employed outsourcing to streamline operations and improve the efficiency of their organizations. However, there is a certain reluctance in the health care industry to employ a strategy used in manufacturing—albeit successfully. Implementing a planned approach to outsourcing, however, can enable health care organizations, large and small, to concentrate their energies on their core competencies.

Outsourcing in Health Care: The Administrator's Guide prepares management to make informed decisions about outsourcing clinical and nonclinical services. The book guides readers through the whole process: developing a strategy for outsourcing; identifying services, functions, and departments that may be outsourced effectively; assessing the potential impact of outsourcing; selecting vendors; preparing requests for proposals and contracts; managing outsourcing relationships; and monitoring vendor performance.

Chapter 1 discusses corporate and health care outsourcing, the trends driving outsourcing, and its potential benefits. In chapter 2, the process of identifying the distinctive competencies of an organization is discussed, as well as the rationale for selecting certain activities for potential outsourcing. Chapters 3, 4, and 5 provide useful information and forms for conducting assessments, setting performance criteria, and developing baseline projections. Chapter 6 details the process of identifying vendors or potential partners. Chapter 7 outlines the process of writing a request for proposal, and chapter 8 presents the key elements of a well-written contract. Chapter 9 defines the role of contract facilitator, and chapter 10 discusses the relevance of effective communication before and during the outsourcing process. Chapter 11 reviews new initiatives, including cosourcing, insourcing, and returning outsourced departments to in-house control.

Administrators may use this book to gain a practical knowledge of the process, then refer to it as they progress through the steps of outsourcing. Managers also may benefit from information that is specific to their role. All readers can clarify their understanding of outsourcing, its benefits and limitations, and how it can serve their health care organizations.

P A R T

I

Introduction

1
Introduction to Outsourcing

Outsourcing is the process of contracting an outside company to provide a service previously performed by staff. In many cases, outsourcing involves a transfer of management responsibility for delivery of service and internal staffing patterns to an outside organization. Subcontracting, contracting out, staff augmentation, flexible staffing, employee leasing, professional services, contract programming, consulting, and contract services are all terms that refer to outsourcing.

This chapter provides an overview of outsourcing, identifies trends driving its growth, and describes its key benefits. A case study on the development and structure of a center of excellence that includes an outsourced component is also presented.

GROWTH OF OUTSOURCING

For decades, health care organizations have outsourced services such as food service and housekeeping. Today, as managed care programs attempt to reduce health care costs, providers are turning to outsourcing in new ways in an effort to maintain high standards of care while addressing current economic realities.

Outsourcing in the Corporate World

Two-thirds of the corporate CEOs surveyed in 1995 as part of *Modern Healthcare*'s annual management survey believed that expertise available to their organizations through outsourcing was valuable and cost-effective.[1]

The corporate world increasingly uses outsourcing to remain competitive. Ross Perot played a key role in the growth of outsourcing when he began offering contracted information systems (IS) to his business clients. Today, IS services are commonly outsourced in business, but no facet of a business is off limits for outsourcing. According to a 1992 survey conducted by A. T. Kearny, Inc., a management consulting firm, 86 percent of the top corporations outsourced services such as payroll, security, uniforms, and food. This was up from 58 percent five years previously.[2]

In recent years, there has been a change in the way major corporations view outsourcing. It has become a significant element in the business planning of most major corporations for strategic, rather than tactical, reasons. Although many corporations are still using outsourcing as a way to reduce costs and substitute for poor internal resource planning, others use it as a way to improve business focus, access new capabilities, and free valuable resources to pursue new ideas.

In a nutshell, corporations are outsourcing for three reasons:

- To focus on core business
- To reduce costs
- To access expertise not available in-house

Outsourcing in the Health Care Industry

Like most other industries, health care is also realizing the advantages of the judicious use of outsourcing. According to *Modern Healthcare*'s 1996 survey of contract management companies, "nearly every category of the top 20 outsourcing areas in hospitals registered at least double-digit gains." Contract management firms reported that their total number of contracts increased 46 percent from 1995 to 1996.[3]

In many ways, health care is becoming like other industries. Administrators do not have the time or personnel to micromanage every department in their organization. When outsourcing is properly executed, health care organizations can use it to parlay existing resources into competitive advantages. By drawing on the expertise and efficiency of vendors who are specialists in their fields, they can free internal management and resources from providing basic services to focusing on the development of superior capabilities in areas that are critical to their future survival and growth.

TRENDS DRIVING THE GROWTH OF OUTSOURCING IN HEALTH CARE

Outsourcing is growing in response to trends in the industry that are changing the way administrators view their organizations. Health care facilities are considering outsourcing as a possible response to demands created by such factors as market pressures, requirements of managed care organizations (MCOs), mergers and acquisitions, and competition within the industry.

Moreover, outsourcing seems to facilitate flexibility at a time when change seems to be the only constant. The structure of health care organizations is evolving as they shed the role of providing all services to providing only carefully selected clinical services. The emerging structure consists of a network of services that are performed by entities that operate as autonomous units with greater maneuverability and adaptability than those held by a more bureaucratic, monolithic entity. This structure greatly increases an organization's ability to respond to continual change.

Market Pressures

Health care organizations that would not have considered outsourcing any services in the past, except those traditionally outsourced such as food and housekeeping, are now considering all non-core competencies for outsourcing. Whereas contracting for traditionally outsourced services is increasing, contracting for clinical services is growing even faster, as evidenced by the following example.

> After Stephen Steinmann went straight through four years of undergraduate work, four years of medical school, and three years of residency in emergency medicine without a break, he graduated from medical school in New Orleans, Louisiana. While Dr. Steinmann was working to earn his credentials, the health care industry was changing rapidly. Hospitals were becoming increasingly reluctant to hire permanent staff. So, after graduation, Dr. Steinmann felt that he needed to travel and explore his options before looking for a permanent position. That's when he turned to the growing *locum tenens* industry to assist him in securing a short-term assignment.

Meanwhile, the administration of a small-town hospital north of San Francisco also contacted a *locum tenens* agency to fill a temporary need for an emergency department physician. The agency recruited Dr. Steinmann, who is board-certified, to be interviewed for the position and carefully checked his credentials. After a full review of the agency report, the hospital, the agency, and Dr. Steinmann agreed that his temporary appointment as emergency department physician was a good move. Dr. Steinmann signed a contract for six months, the agency covered the cost of malpractice insurance, and the hospital paid for plane fare and Dr. Steinmann's apartment.

This outsourcing agreement gave the hospital the expertise it needed in the emergency department without the long-term commitment of hiring a full-time employee. The hospital is now conducting a feasibility study to determine whether there would be significant cost savings in contracting out the management of the entire emergency department. Approximately 50 percent of hospitals hire contract management firms to manage their emergency departments.[4]

Requirements of Managed Care Organizations

With the growth of managed care, failure to develop a plan for forming relationships with MCOs puts health care organizations at risk of losing market share. However, entering into managed care contracts without carefully considering all aspects of service delivery is equally risky.

Health care organizations need to define their roles in provider networks and decide if they want to assume responsibility for the full continuum of care dictated by MCOs or to contract with others to fill gaps in their existing array of services. Creating a continuum of care while simultaneously keeping costs down may necessitate establishing relationships with other providers. Therefore, it is important for hospitals considering MCO membership to devise a plan for establishing relationships with contractors capable of delivering the seamless web of services required by managed care. In 1995, *Forbes* reported that OrNda, a major hospital company in southern Florida, southern California, Arizona/Nevada, and other states, intended to be "a kind of wholesaler of services" for health maintenance organizations. By using outsourcing to offer the spectrum of services required by MCOs, this for-profit hospital chain chose to capitalize on the MCO trend.[5]

This philosophy has led to growth particularly in the outsourcing of imaging services. Two forces have combined to create the need for outsourcing imaging services, especially computer tomography (CT) and magnetic resonance imaging (MRI): physicians and their patients are demanding the latest imaging technology, and MCOs want these services to control costs. Therefore, small- or medium-size hospitals are increasingly likely to search for ways to avoid making the huge capital investments required for MRI and CT technology. The answer may lie in outsourcing these services.

> In New Hampshire, six trailers carrying MRI machines travel around the state. The trailers park in the hospitals' parking lots and attach to hospitals with an air lock like the ones used at airports. Another high-tech mobile unit, a $2 million lithotripter, which is used to break up kidney stones with sound waves, also travels the scenic roads of New Hampshire.[6] This mobile technology serves the needs of patients while saving the hospitals the huge capital investment that would be necessary if it were not for their outsourcing contracts.

Mergers and Acquisitions

The record number of mergers and acquisitions in the health care industry is also contributing to the growth of outsourcing. During a merger, individual hospital facilities may find themselves in competition with other providers in the new organization. Therefore, they must develop an individual identity separate from, but complementary to, the other members. In this way, although mergers can be disruptive, they may also provide an opportunity for organizational transformation. Some hospitals may develop centers of excellence in product lines such as coronary care, while others develop their obstetrics department. Thus, a merger provides an opportunity for growth fueled by a reduction in the costs of competition.

Moreover, mergers force an evaluation of information services. The need for a shared database, elimination of duplicate services, and the complexity of a large integrated system may exceed internal IS expertise and capabilities. IS outsourcing can provide the cutting-edge skills required by merging health care systems. Highly skilled IS professionals are indispensable when the transition to a consolidated system is at its peak; however, many of them will be unnecessary when the system is established. Therefore, outsourcing fills the temporary need of the hospital for IS expertise that will keep it competitive, while avoiding the dilemma of hiring workers only to lay them off after the transition period. Also, IS outsourcing during a merger can prevent conflict over which computer system to adopt. Each hospital IS executive will argue to retain his or her system and convert the others. By functioning objectively, the outside company can serve to defuse this potentially divisive situation.

Competition

Large competitors may be stable enough not to suffer severe losses from a merger in their market areas, although they are certain to lose some revenue share to new centers of excellence that will be trumpeted by the emerging health care network. However, small competitors will find it difficult to compete with the economies of scale realized by newly merged hospitals. They may respond by seeking to merge with a larger facility or by pursuing managed care contracts. Or they may focus their efforts on a limited number of areas, while using the expertise of outside firms to fill gaps in the continuum of care required by MCOs. Indeed, outsourcing contracts such as these may prove to be their salvation.

BENEFITS OF OUTSOURCING

Outsourcing can support both market maneuvers and core competencies. *Market maneuvers* are strategic initiatives implemented to take advantage of market conditions. A *core competency*, also called *distinctive competency*, is a highly focused mixture of skills and technologies that make it possible for a company to produce services of value.

Market Maneuvers

In a constantly changing market, health care administrators can use outsourcing to increase their flexibility and respond to market opportunities as they occur. Outsourcing can also reduce the problems associated with fluctuating staffing needs. Market maneuvers can be more successfully implemented when providers and vendors share risks and benefits, which can be accomplished in the following ways:

- *Flexible planning:* Outsourcing allows health care organizations to be flexible in planning and to focus on initiatives quickly. Providers must anticipate the changing market and respond. For instance, outpatient care is expected to account for nearly 50 percent of net patient revenues by the year 2000.[7] Outsourcing may be used to supply outpatient diagnostic services if the provider has planned for this change.
- *Elimination of peak staffing problems:* Outsourcing a service for which the demand fluctuates dramatically can eliminate the need to carry full-time employees during low-demand times while still offering adequate staffing during peak-demand periods.
- *Risk and benefit sharing:* Health care organizations may create partnerships with vendors in which the risk of the new services will be shared. In this way, both parties will be committed to the hard work it takes to create a successful partnership, and both will benefit.

Core Competencies

Health care administrators can focus more efficiently on their distinctive competencies by allowing vendors to deal with day-to-day administration, relieving them of the constant demand to make decisions and respond to a barrage of issues competing for attention. Moreover, outsourcing can free resources that can then be directed to enhancing and supporting core competencies. This can be accomplished through the following:

- *Acquisition of technical expertise:* Some departments with rapidly changing technology, such as radiology, require high levels of technical expertise from their personnel. Technical experts can help administrators make the best decisions about equipment acquisition so that the department can remain current.

- *A focus on excellence:* Many executives believe that companies can benefit from outsourcing because the vendor is focused on maintaining expertise in its specific area.
- *Cost reduction:* Cost reduction may result from outsourcing because the outside contractor usually will have lower costs as a result of economies of scale. Some outsourcing arrangements also eliminate internal administrative and maintenance costs and free facility space that can be used more profitably.
- *Reduction of capital requirements:* By outsourcing support services, the organization can redirect the capital required for such purchases as imaging or movable medical equipment.

CREATING A CENTER OF EXCELLENCE: A CASE STUDY

A large urban hospital had always been known as a maternity hospital, drawing patients from a metropolitan area of three million people. As the birth rate declined and malpractice rates soared, administrators reevaluated the necessity for its obstetrics department.

The administration conducted a public survey and an internal analysis, which revealed that obstetrics was essential to the identity of the hospital. It was found that the department also brought new patients to the hospital who continued on to use pediatric and other services. Therefore, the administrators decided to enhance and promote this distinctive competency. In the face of declining birth rates in its catchment area, this hospital decided to create a center of excellence for women's health. To house the center, designers transformed unused square footage created by shorter hospital stays and excess storage space brought about by the use of the hospital's new "just-in-time" materials management system.

First, the hospital decided to enhance its already excellent obstetrics department. Six new midwifery practitioners joined the existing practice of three nurse midwives. Meanwhile, the hospital continued birthing classes and chose to make a capital investment in five new birthing suites. In addition, a search committee recruited a prominent expert from a competing local hospital to head the genetic testing and counseling unit.

Next, the hospital created an outpatient treatment and education center for women. The women's center offered parenting classes, sibling classes, and women's health classes. In response to the needs identified through focus groups, the center included a state-of-the-art mammography center adjacent to the OB/GYN examining rooms and a small women's health library in the center of the lobby/waiting area. In addition, counseling on topics such as nutrition, birth control, and menopause was offered, an exercise studio held classes and individualized training consultations, and a child care center was provided nearby.

The new women's center also sought the expertise of outside lactation consultants, who had already established a reputation for excellence within the community. By signing an outsourcing contract with these consultants, the new women's center was able to achieve immediate excellence in this area and a positive reputation, eliminating the time and expense of the learning curve that would have been required by internal staff development.

Marketing and public relations campaigns emphasized the comprehensive services offered at the new women's center, and the hospital's external affairs office created posters and brochures presenting the women's center as an umbrella organization for all of women's health concerns. Free public lectures focusing on current research into health issues of concern to women were held at the center. Media coverage generated by these events attracted the attention of women from all over the metropolitan area. In time, the women's center became a valuable community resource, and the hospital strengthened its already excellent reputation.

CONCLUSION

A general understanding of outsourcing and how it can support goals and strategies is important to a successful health care organization. Outsourcing, the process of contracting with an outside company to supply services, can be used to support distinctive competencies or to take advantage of market conditions. The increased use of outsourcing in the health care industry is a response to market trends. After exploring the impact of market trends on their particular situation, administrators will be prepared to evaluate the potential benefits of outsourcing functions that may be distracting attention and funding from more lucrative activities. For these administrators, subsequent chapters in this book will provide a step-by-step approach to the process of outsourcing.

References

1.   J. D. Moore, Jr. Outsiders on the Inside Track; *Modern Healthcare*'s Annual Contract Management Survey Shows Hospitals Finding More Reasons to Opt against In-house Expertise, *Modern Healthcare* (September 1996): 67.

2.   G. S. Johnson. When Only Hired Guns Will Do; Survey: More Fortune 100 Firms Outsourcing Company Activities, *Journal of Commerce and Commercial* 409, no. 1 (28759) (July 1996): 3B.

3.   S. Hensley. Outsourcing Boom: Survey Shows More Hospitals Turning to Outside Firms for a Broad Range of Services, *Modern Healthcare* (September 1997): 51.

4.   J. Greene. Contracts Are Catching On, *Modern Healthcare* (January 1994): 29.

5.   R. Koselka. Babies Are Welcome, *Forbes* 155, no. 9 (April 1995): 144–50.

6.   B. Sanders. "Outsourcing" Gives Hospitals Technology without the Costs, *New Hampshire Business Review* 18, no. 7 (March 1996): 7A.

7.   J. Surpin. Hospitals Enhance Their Capacities for Change, *Health Care Competition Week* (January 1993).

An Outsourcing Model

2

Conducting a Strategic Analysis

Outsourcing is a step-by-step process that is applied to increase effectiveness and efficiency. The first step in this process is to conduct a strategic analysis. A strategic analysis is an analysis of an organization's resources and capabilities to identify strengths and weaknesses. The strategic analysis provides a foundation for making decisions about priorities, identifying distinctive competencies that should *not* be outsourced, and selecting internal candidates for outsourcing.

This chapter discusses outsourcing as a strategic tool. It describes the two strategic reasons why a health care organization might decide to outsource and outlines a method for conducting a strategic analysis of the organization's outsourcing needs.

OUTSOURCING AS A STRATEGIC TOOL

The process of strategic outsourcing requires executive direction because it involves changes in the strategy, structure, and staffing of the organization. Thus, outsourcing must be driven from the top. Before engaging in outsourcing, managers must understand and carry out the process of strategic analysis—clarifying the goals of the organization, identifying its distinctive competencies, and selecting internal departments, services, or functions as candidates for outsourcing.

Outsourcing plays an important role in helping health care organizations pursue strategic intent by forcing them to identify and enhance their distinctive competencies, thus bringing vision of purpose into focus. An organization should develop and maintain a balance between its vision and its resources. To turn vision into reality, the organization must develop its economic resources. Strategic outsourcing, then, can provide the wherewithal for fulfilling this vision by reducing overall costs and freeing existing resources so they can be used to enhance distinctive competencies that most clearly define the organization's role in the health care community.

Development of a Strategic Plan

The process of strategic outsourcing should begin with a strategic plan. Health care organizations use strategic plans to ensure consistency in decision making and to allocate resources effectively and efficiently. A strategic plan presents an analysis of the organization's current situation and charts a formal program for guiding its development in the future. Typically, a strategic plan includes a mission statement that defines the organization's primary purpose for existence, objectives reflecting its mission, goals for specific areas, and tactics for achieving those goals. The plan also addresses various market forces that can affect the success of the health care operation over time. The plan involves prioritization of capital, management direction, and the assignment of responsibilities to employees.[1]

The strategic plan should identify the potential role of outsourcing in achieving the organization's objectives and set specific goals for areas to be outsourced. In addition, the plan should evaluate whether current vendors can meet the organization's objectives, anticipate operational or organizational shifts, and identify future needs effectively. Finally, it should outline specific steps that must be taken to accomplish the goals of outsourcing and provide detailed information for annual capital planning.

Strategic Reasons for Outsourcing

There are two primary strategic reasons for outsourcing: to improve focus on distinctive competencies and to achieve competitive differentiation.

Improving Focus on Distinctive Competencies.   Health care organizations should identify areas of expertise that are intrinsic to the success of their institutions and retain control of them. Therefore, it is important to separate vital services that must be provided in-house from less critical services that may be contracted to suppliers. For example, if a facility is focused on cancer care, it does not make sense to outsource services related to oncology, such as radiation therapy. Conversely, radiation therapy may be an appropriate area for outsourcing for a pediatric hospital.

By allowing outside vendors to assume responsibility for the nitty-gritty details of a variety of everyday operational activities, outsourcing frees internal resources so that the health care organization can continue to refine and improve its distinctive competencies. Companies such as the pharmaceutical giant Merck have demonstrated success in building strategies around core competencies and outsourcing as many other activities as possible. As a result, Merck has created a less integrated, but more focused, organization. Health care facilities can also tighten their operations by delegating the performance of a service, department, or function to an outside vendor so they can free their resources to develop their own distinctive niche in the health care community.

Responding to Market Opportunities.   Outsourcing makes it possible for health care administrators to respond more rapidly to market changes that affect their organizations. By reducing direct day-to-day responsibility for certain functions through outsourcing, administrators are more likely to respond to changing market forces by initiating new projects. For example, the shorter hospital stays dictated by MCOs have created surplus hospital beds. This market force, in combination with a dramatic growth in the elderly population, has prompted some health care organizations to convert these empty beds to skilled or long-term care, thus providing a dual hospital/nursing home function.[2-4] Recognition of such an opportunity becomes more likely when administrators are not encumbered with responsibility for everyday services that may be handled by an outside vendor.

To identify market opportunities that could be enhanced by outsourcing, hospital administrators should respond to the following questions regarding those departments, services, or functions they plan to outsource:

- Does this activity respond to the needs of the community?
- Is it an appropriate focus in the current health care market?
- Is utilization commensurate with the demographics of the service area?

- How is this activity rated on patient satisfaction surveys?
- Are there any indications of how the community would feel about an outsourced service?
- How is the vendor perceived?
- How is the service perceived? (For example, the community may hold a different impression of geriatrics than of pediatrics.)
- Does the organization wish to obtain specialized expertise or access to advanced technology?

STEP-BY-STEP METHOD FOR CONDUCTING A STRATEGIC ANALYSIS

A strategic analysis should be conducted before a health care organization embarks on outsourcing. The first step in conducting this analysis is to form a planning team and an operations team. The planning team works primarily on defining and carrying out the organization's vision, and the operations team defines goals and identifies candidates for outsourcing. After these teams are in place, the organization next defines its goals, identifies its distinctive competencies, and classifies and evaluates candidates (services, functions, or departments) for outsourcing.

Forming a Planning Team

As an integral part of the strategic analysis, the planning team must involve a collaboration of administrators, planners, and managers who can develop a vision of how the health care organization should be organized and operated. The vision is part of the organization's strategic plan, discussed earlier. In some circumstances, the planning team may include members of the organization's board of trustees. If there is an annual planning retreat, the planning team may want to take advantage of its insights concerning the long-term prospects of the organization.

Forming an Operations Team

After the planning team has performed its analysis, the administration should appoint an operations team. This team will be called on to clarify organizational goals, define distinctive competencies, delineate the goals of outsourcing, and identify appropriate candidates for outsourcing by projecting their economic value and examining their intrinsic necessity to the success of the organization.

The operations team should involve participants from materials management, finance, planning, nursing, administration, human resources, legal, and communications. Other members of the staff, such as department heads and physicians, may be involved during specific steps of the outsourcing process. Although staff members are knowledgeable and experienced in operating health care institutions, they are generally not experienced in evaluating, negotiating, and managing outsourcing contracts; therefore, the in-house team may be complemented by outside planners and contract facilitators.

Identifying Distinctive Competencies

As a rule, organizations should not outsource distinctive competencies that are intrinsic to their success. Most health care organizations choose to outsource carefully selected activities that can be accomplished more quickly, for less cost, and more effectively by outside resources. Therefore, it is essential to identify distinctive competencies in order to retain control of those areas by internal staff.

Health care organizations may identify distinctive competencies by examining two dimensions of each service or department: organizational strength (figure 2-1) and market appeal (figure 2-2). For example, a nursing home with excellent indicators for dealing with skin breakdown and a reputation for positive public perceptions would not consider outsourcing wound care. Conversely, an outpatient radiology center with unacceptable throughput and significant levels of competition would not be acting prudently if it attempted to develop a women's health screening program internally. Health care organizations will realize the greatest returns from efforts invested in programs in which they have demonstrated strengths and that attract market attention.

In identifying distinctive competencies, the outsourcing team may review the following questions:

- Is this activity intrinsic to the identity of the health care organization?

FIGURE 2-1.   Indicators of Quality/Organizational Strength for (Department, Service, or Function)

	Excellent	Acceptable	Needs Improvement	Unacceptable
Calculate mortality rate by diagnosis				
Calculate readmission rate by diagnosis >30 days >60 days >90 days				
Calculate morbidity rate by diagnosis				
Calculate ALOS by diagnosis				
Calculate complication rate by diagnosis				
Calculate compliance with treatment protocols				
Facilities				
General appearance				
Furnishings				
Signage				
Equipment				
Inventory (number of pieces)				
Technology				
Efficiency				
Calculate throughput				
Calculate utilization				
Financial				
Calculate savings of resources				
Calculate return on investment				
Revenue enhancement				

FIGURE 2-2. Indicators of Market Appeal for (Department, Service, or Function)

	Excellent	Acceptable	Needs Improvement	Unacceptable
Reimbursement mix and coverage				
Degree of regulation				
Competition				
Market share				
Market growth				
Market				
Knowledge				
Positioning				
Image				
Identity program				
Patient complaints				
Referral channels				
Public perception of care				

- How does this activity differentiate this health care system from its competitors?
- Does this activity provide a strategic or competitive advantage?
- Which services are too critical to entrust to a vendor?
- Is this service a component of the organization's strategic thrust?

Defining Goals for Outsourcing

Accurate, pertinent information on the health care organization's strategic advantages is the cornerstone of successful outsourcing. The operations team should review the organization's position in the current market before setting goals. Answering the following questions may help:

- How large is the territory covered by your market?
- How is your market structured? Is it scattered? Are there important segments?

- What are the important segments?
- What are the demographics, use of services, and attitude of each segment?
- What percentage of your market uses third-party payers? What are their attitudes and operations?
- What are the effects of the following on your market: Age? Income? Occupation? Increasing population? Decreasing birth rate?
- What is the organization's image?
- What are the components of that image?

The next critical step for the operations team is to identify precise goals for outsourcing (for example, reduce cost, improve processes, and/or enhance customer satisfaction).

Some questions to consider when setting objectives and goals for outsourcing are:

- How does current staffing for the activity considered for outsourcing compare with other health care systems?
- Do quality indicators for this service fall below external benchmarks for similar services?
- What impact will outsourcing have on employees and internal culture?
- What capital investments will be needed over the next five years?

Identifying Candidates for Outsourcing

The operations team next identifies departments and services best suited to outsourcing and sets priorities for the utilization of existing and potential resources to strengthen the organization's position in the health care community. Any area of an organization that is not a distinctive competency can be considered for outsourcing. From a purely practical standpoint, three areas may be outsourced—departments, services, and functions. Each of these areas can be divided into health care and non-health care activities. (See figure 2-3.)

These areas offer many opportunities for outsourcing. One of the most difficult tasks at this stage is identifying candidates that represent opportunities to exert the greatest influence on the future of the health care organization. To identify the best candidates for outsourcing, it is necessary to list areas that do not provide distinctive competencies and

FIGURE 2-3. Three Areas of Outsourcing Contracts

	Service	Department	Function
Non-health care examples	Equipment Maintenance Security	Dietary Linen Food services	Transportation Materials management Accounting
Health care examples	CT scanning Social services Visiting nurses	Physical therapy Radiology Emergency	Asset management Planning Insurance

then determine return on investment for outsourcing those areas. Asking certain questions might assist in clarifying those candidates best suited to outsourcing, such as:

- Does this activity generate revenue?
- Is the revenue generated higher or lower than the expense associated with the activity?
- Will future changes in reimbursement affect this activity?
- Does the acquisition/merger plan directly affect this activity?
- Does this service add significant value to the quality of health care delivered?
- Does the organization require significant capital investment in order to maintain or improve performance?
- Has this service suffered from poor performance (financial or qualitative) in the past?
- Are there contracts and/or service agreements related to this service that will expire in the next 12 to 18 months?
- Does this service have significant fluctuations in utilization?
- Does the supply of qualified labor for this service vary significantly over time?

Outsourcing Services and Departments.   Outsourcing a service involves assigning administrative responsibility for a specific activity, usually within one department, to a third party. Outsourcing a department involves turning an entire department over to the vendor. The outsourcing of services, such as food service, security, housekeeping, and even patient care facilities like the emergency department, is common and familiar; however, the outsourcing of functions deserves further attention.

Outsourcing Functions.   Outsourcing a function involves segregating an activity that crosses departmental lines and assigning it to the vendor.

Functions are typically more difficult to define and segregate than services or departments. A number of people may share a function, either as an official responsibility or as an assumed role. For instance, ordering supplies may involve numerous individuals in an institution. The purchasing department has official responsibility for external purchases, while the warehouse or central supply staff is responsible for internal purchases or deliveries. However, interviews with staff may reveal that a number of people throughout the institution participate in that function.

Whether it is the nurse who orders extra supplies, the aide who tells the sales representative that more product is needed, or the manager who approves a shipment, each has assumed a responsibility in the supply ordering process. They may have done so because they feel they have a better understanding of the needs of their department, or they may have encountered a problem obtaining supplies in the past. Whatever the reason, these distractions will have a negative impact on their ability to do their own jobs. Outsourcing all materials management purchasing functions should eliminate duplicate efforts and streamline the process.

For example, a 500-bed urban hospital reorganized its transportation services by outsourcing the movement of supplies, equipment, records, drugs, and other objects to one company; outsourcing the movement of patients to another; and handling the transport of clinical specimens internally by installing a pneumatic tube system. These changes allowed for a reduction in full-time employees, streamlined a number of systems, and increased efficiency.

Candidates for outsourcing should be classified and evaluated according to their relative importance in affecting distinctive competencies and strategic initiatives of the health care organization. Figure 2-4 presents a framework that may be used to classify services, departments, and functions in terms of their relative importance in fulfilling strategic intent and contributing economic value to the health care system. Services that do not support distinctive competencies should be considered for outsourcing before services that do.

OUTSOURCING A SUPPORT FUNCTION: A CASE STUDY

A three-hospital system wanted to develop plans to better integrate the three facilities and partner with other facilities and systems. While the

FIGURE 2-4. Framework for Classifying Outsourcing Candidates

How does this department, service, or function contribute to:

Hospital Identity (Distinctive)
- Defines organization (e.g., radiation therapy department in a hospital with a cancer center)

Performance
- Drives daily performance (e.g., translating department in a hospital with numerous non-English-speaking patients)

Overhead
- Supports other activities (e.g., telecommunications center)

Legal Mandate
- Compliance with governmental regulations (e.g., radiation safety)

Culture
- Conducted because of tradition (e.g., pastoral services)

Economic Value
- Produces positive or economically neutral cash flow (e.g., coffee shop)

Strategic Impact
- Essential to the identity or functional capacity of the organization (e.g., mobile mammography in a rural health clinic)

planning staff at the individual hospitals had been adept at developing strategic courses for their own organizations, they had not been able to develop a comprehensive view of the system. Then, the corporate vice-president of planning announced her departure.

The president and his key advisors believed that the planning position was key to the future prosperity of the system. However, there did not appear to be any viable candidates to fill the position internally. Finally, the group decided that instead of trying to replace the vice-president of planning, they would approach outside firms that had the ability to perform strategic planning.

Three firms were contacted. One declined consideration because a contract with a competitor constituted a potential conflict of interest. The other two firms were asked to submit proposals outlining a plan and listing references from similar projects. This process eliminated another firm. The planning staff was pleased with the response offered by the third firm and signed a contract with them. As a result, several positions were eliminated and the planning staff was consolidated.

During the next nine months, the planning firm conducted both an internal and an external assessment, identifying strengths, weaknesses, opportunities, and threats (SWOT). A plan that identified internal steps that should be taken and potential affiliations was prepared. Implementation of this plan resulted in increased efficiency within the system as well as a merger with another system. The latter gave the combined system market leadership in its region.

Many organizations would shy away from outsourcing a function as critical as planning. However, provided adequate internal monitoring and control, it may be no more risky than outsourcing other departments. The purpose of outsourcing is to refocus efforts on core elements while letting others with more expertise handle nonessential functions. When outsourcing an area with few quantifiable indicators, the monitoring function becomes even more critical. The key is to develop mileposts by which to measure the vendor's performance. In this example, mileposts might have included completion of the SWOT analysis, development of an internal plan, and identification of appropriate merger partners.

Here are some recommendations to consider before outsourcing strategic planning:

- Contact several vendors and make a choice based on positive feedback from other clients as well as on cost issues.
- Develop a time line for completion of this project and incorporate it into the contract with the vendor.
- Develop mileposts by which to measure vendor performance.
- Identify areas of opportunity that the external firm should investigate for the future.
- Determine how long the arrangement will continue.

CONCLUSION

It is easier for an organization to build on its strengths than to shore up its weaknesses. Health care organizations should develop strengths that lie in areas in which they can outperform their competitors. Rather than rely on perceptions, they should go through a disciplined process of strategic analysis that distinguishes distinctive competencies from other activities. By identifying strengths, health care organizations can pursue opportunities and goals in areas that match their competencies.

References

1. P. G. Keen and E. M. Knapp. *Every Manager's Guide to Business Processes* (Boston: Harvard Business School Press, 1995), p. 183.

2. Geriatrics Is Especially Well-Suited to Outsourcing. Here's Why, *Hospitals and Health Networks* 70, no. 9 (May 1996): 36.

3. J. D. Moore, Jr. Outsiders on the Inside Track: *Modern Healthcare's* Annual Contract Management Survey Shows Hospitals Finding More Reasons to Opt against In-house Expertise, *Modern Healthcare* (September 1996): 67.

4. T. T. Rice. Cast Me Not Off in the Time of Age, *Hospitals and Health Networks* 70, no. 9 (May 1996): 34–38.

3

Performing an Outsourcing Assessment

After the operations committee has determined the role that outsourcing will play in the health care organization's competitive positioning and growth, a formal outsourcing assessment must be conducted to determine the current performance levels of the organization's various departments or services and to identify any problems or gaps in services. Conducting an outsourcing assessment helps to define requirements to be supplied by vendors and prepares organizations to match requirements for services to be outsourced with current needs, rather than historical performance.

This chapter divides the outsourcing assessment process into two principal functions: collecting the data and analyzing them to identify performance gaps. It also offers a case study of a health care organization that decided to outsource its equipment repairs.

COLLECTING THE DATA

Evaluating whether a department, service, or function is a candidate for outsourcing can provide information on organizational structure and routines and point out operational or staffing inefficiencies. An assessment should define the mission (if a department), evaluate service, identify customers, and uncover problems.

A team approach to performing an assessment works best. The operations team should assign assessment activities to subgroups consisting of team members. In the case of a departmental assessment, one group might concentrate on how the department functions internally; a second group might examine its effect on other areas and customers; and a third group, with input from the department manager, might perform an analysis of department expenses.

Some questions to ask during formal assessment are:

- What does this function/department contribute to the organization?
- How efficient is function/department performance?
- What costs are associated with this department or activity?
- Will outsourcing this activity/department have any negative impact?
- What does the competition do in this area?
- What impact will outsourcing have internally on employees, physicians, and other departments or services?
- What impact will outsourcing have externally on insurers, patients, suppliers, and other members of the community?
- Are similar activities performed by other departments in the organization?
- Are these activities accomplished more efficiently there?
- How satisfied are their "customers"?
- Can this activity be separated from other functions so that it might be considered for outsourcing?
- Does this activity have the potential to add value to the organization or to any specific product lines, now or in the future?

The formal assessment process includes:

- Developing flowcharts for each department/service/function to be reviewed
- Preparing a financial assessment on the impact of outsourcing
- Conducting interviews to identify current perceptions of satisfaction, quality, and morale

Developing Flowcharts

A simple flowchart is a useful tool for defining the specific tasks that are carried out by each service or department. It can be used to identify key relationships, determine internal flaws, and develop corrective procedures. A flowchart documents every step of an activity from start to finish, noting how decisions are made and responsibilities designated. (See figure 3-1.)

FIGURE 3-1. Sample Flowchart

Physician order → Telephone request to Central Distribution → Is item available?

Is item available? — Yes → Central Distribution delivers item → Item placed on patient → Patient charge generated → Stop

Is item available? — No → Are there other items unused on the nursing unit?

Are there other items unused on the nursing unit? — Yes → Nurse picks up item from other nursing unit → Item placed on patient

Are there other items unused on the nursing unit? — No → Nurses telephone other nursing units → Are there other items unused on the nursing unit?

Are there other items unused on the nursing unit? — Yes → Nurse obtains item and cleans → Nurse picks up item from other nursing unit

Are there other items unused on the nursing unit? — No → Are there any patients who do not need the item?

Are there any patients who do not need the item? — Yes → Nurse obtains item and cleans

Are there any patients who do not need the item? — No → Notify physician of problem

After a flowchart has been created, the next step is to analyze the process or flow to determine how an activity can be improved, isolated, or segregated so that it can be either made more productive or targeted for outsourcing. For example, as figure 3-1 shows, when equipment is unavailable, finding the item becomes the responsibility of the nursing staff—an inefficient and wasteful process. The operations team can evaluate this problem to determine whether internal intervention or outsourcing is the most appropriate solution to the problem of finding needed equipment.

Preparing a Financial Assessment

A financial assessment identifies all costs associated with a department, function, or service. To determine true costs, the budget, the income and expense statement, and the indirect costs of overhead, such as distribution, administrative support, and planning, all should be examined. "Assigning indirect costs on the basis of the resources consumed by specific products or services requires a detailed analysis of the relevant activities and cost structures," according to Keen and Knapp's business process guide.[1]

To avoid the confusion associated with intermingling hard and soft costs, the financial analysis should separate these two categories. Hard costs are defined as those that have a direct impact on the institution's financial statements, including direct salary expenses, lease payments, and supply costs. Soft costs, on the other hand, may prove more difficult to factor into consideration during the financial analysis, because they have a less direct impact on finances. Examples of soft costs are the time spent by nurses looking for medical equipment or messengers delivering lab reports. Eliminating these tasks may improve efficiency; however, rarely will the number of full-time-equivalent employees be reduced.

Conducting Interviews

Through interviews with hospital administrators, department heads, and key physicians, it is possible to obtain new information about operational and functional requirements. Interviews, which can be done in person or by questionnaire, are valuable because they can:

- Build consensus by involving the staff in the planning process. When staff members participate, they know they have contributed to the plan. Thus, they have a sense of ownership in their department or service.
- Provide insights into the staff's understanding of the future volume of business and staffing requirements.
- Identify each department's or service's primary customer as patient or physician.
- Analyze the perceived quality of services provided.
- Validate the information obtained in the flowcharting process through interviews with internal customers that can highlight both positive and negative aspects of each department or service, pinpoint potential problem areas, and define expectations.

ANALYZING THE DATA AND IDENTIFYING PERFORMANCE GAPS

The data gathered during the assessment phase must now be analyzed. The goal is to compare the actual operation of the department/service/function with the expectations of the customers, as gathered during the interview process. Questions that might be considered are:

- Does the department/service/function meet the needs of its customers?
- Is it unable to meet basic requirements? If so, what are they?
- Have the customers found methods to overcome or circumvent the deficiencies of the department/service/function? How?

The difference between customer expectations and actual performance is a *performance gap*. Outsourcing should minimize performance gaps. If performance gaps are easily remedied with internal intervention, there may be no need for outsourcing.

The assessment process may uncover facets of an operation that the staff has resolved with a "Band-Aid" approach that falls outside the realm of their normal operating procedures. For example, after patient transportation was outsourced in one hospital, several departments began complaining that expected faxes were never delivered. An investigation revealed that in the past, the patient transport department had maintained a central fax machine and had hand-delivered documents. Because the vendor was unaware of this unofficial activity, faxes were no longer delivered. An analysis of the results of the department interviews might have prevented such problems by providing the team members with a more thorough understanding of department operations.

After the internal activities that customers or patients view as crucial to their satisfaction have been identified and their costs estimated, focus can be directed to key elements that ensure patient satisfaction, curb costs, or improve revenue. At this point, it is time to examine how other organizations have successfully undertaken such tasks. This process, called benchmarking, will be discussed in chapter 4.

REVIEWING THE FINDINGS

In addition to providing information on the way each department, service, or function is handled currently, the interviews often produce ideas from staff members about how a service/function may be conducted (or a department operated) more productively in the future. This information may be of considerable assistance in determining which departments, services, or functions to outsource.

Services that add value to an activity should be maintained; those that detract should be improved or eliminated. This analysis provides a preliminary template of the ideal efficient department, whether it is to be maintained internally or externally. For instance, in organizing the laundry/linen department, colored blankets should continue to be provided if they are frequently mentioned in patient satisfaction surveys. Conversely, if early morning pickup (i.e., 5 A.M.) of soiled linen generates complaints from housekeeping, a new pickup schedule should be considered.

The operations team must now review the findings of the formal assessment, with an eye toward identifying appropriate candidates for outsourcing. From a global viewpoint, those departments/services/ functions that are not critical to the main strategic thrust of the organization should be placed on the candidate list.

Another aspect of performing assessments is that they can reveal those departments/services/functions that require significant investment by the organization to maintain technological standing, such as information systems, laundry, physician office billing, and plant maintenance. The operations team should consider what the desired goal of outsourcing should be: enhanced level of service, cost reduction, elimination of non-core functions, or some combination of these.

OUTSOURCING EQUIPMENT REPAIRS: A CASE STUDY

A 300-bed community hospital was looking for ways to consolidate its operations to enhance efficiency and decrease cost. One area that had been identified as a possible candidate for improvement was equipment maintenance. To perform an audit of this function, a team consisting of the administrator, a staff member from the finance department, and the materials manager developed the assessment tool presented in figure 3-2.

After observing the movement of equipment to and from clinical engineering and the work flow within each department, the team interviewed employees of the departments involved. Using flowchart observations, financial data, and the results of interviews with department managers and staff, the team found that preventive maintenance was delinquent, in-house expertise was lacking, and parts inventory was excessive. For these reasons, it recommended that equipment maintenance be outsourced. The team recommended a two-step process. All equipment except radiology would be outsourced first, because planned equipment acquisitions would limit maintenance requirements for one year. Maintenance of the radiology equipment would be included in the outsourcing in the future.

CONCLUSION

The information gathered in the assessment helps determine whether to redesign the existing department, service, or function, to insource it by assigning it to individuals who have demonstrated excellence within the organization but outside the primary department, or to outsource it.

For example, in its current configuration, a department may not be meeting the needs of internal customers. Problem solving and redesign may be necessary to engender a higher degree of satisfaction by users.

FIGURE 3-2. Assessment Tool for Outsourcing Equipment Repairs

Equipment Type

Respiratory

Neonatal

Operating room

Central distribution lab

Radiology lab

Lab

Critical care

Other

Outsourcing Equipment Maintenance

A. Clinical engineering

   1. Personnel allocation:
      FTEs
      Salary

   2. Hours of operation:

   3. Overtime expenditures:

   4. Parts expenses:

   5. Outside repair expenses:

   6. Average turnaround time on repairs:

   7. Number of pieces of equipment:

   8. Estimated average age of equipment:

   9. Average response time for repairs:

   10. How does equipment get to clinical engineering?

   11. How is equipment returned to the department?

B. Materials management

   1. What equipment maintenance contracts are in place?

   2. What contracts will be expiring and when?

   3. Are there capital requests for equipment? For what and are they approved?

FIGURE 3-2.   (Continued)

C. User departments

    1. Do you use clinical engineering for equipment repairs? Which equipment?

    2. Do you have equipment for which you do not use clinical engineering? What equipment? How is this equipment repaired?

    3. Review the service agreements provided by materials management. Do you have others?

    4. Average response time for repairs:

    5. How does equipment get to clinical engineering?

    6. How is equipment returned to the department?

    7. How satisfied are you with the turnaround time?

    8. Are there improvements you would like to see?

    9. Other comments:

Redesign may require retraining of existing staff, replacement of positions with another level (for example, replacement of certified nursing assistants with registered nurses), separation of jobs, or creation of work groups to resolve problems. Sometimes, capital investment, such as facility renovation or a high-tech purchase, may be necessary.

After the assessment, the health care organization will have a clearer picture of how things work under the current structure. This picture will reveal what is and is not financially profitable and where quality and efficiency may need improvement. Thus, the stage will be set for evaluating these services, departments, and functions in comparison with similar departments in other organizations.

Reference

1. P. G. Keen and E. M. Knapp. *Every Manager's Guide to Business Processes* (Boston: Harvard Business School Press, 1995), p. 40.

4

Setting Performance Criteria

The outsourcing assessment described in chapter 3 comes into play during the request for proposal (RFP) phase, when vendors submit a detailed explanation of what and how they will perform the activity to be outsourced. (See chapter 7.) It is also used after an outsourcing contract has been implemented as a way to accurately assess the level of service provided by the vendor. Some health care organizations skip this step and later find they have no mechanism to determine if the activity is being performed at the desired level. This pitfall can be avoided by setting and monitoring performance criteria.

This chapter discusses how to identify performance indicators, how to choose appropriate indicators, and how to compare internal indicators with external benchmarks. Benchmarking is the calibration of an organization's performance against the performance achieved by others in the field. A case study at the back of the chapter illustrates how benchmarks were applied in a health care organization that provides subacute care.

THE PROCESS

The customer (patient, physician, or payer) can be used to help identify areas needing improvement. Key activities or tasks that define the level of performance expected by the customer should be identified. Examples might include turnaround time on patient equipment requests (where the customer is the nurse), the number of errors on a patient bill (where the customer is the payer), and the wait time to schedule an operative procedure (where the customer is the physician). A more complete list appears in figure 4-1. The key concern is to develop a list of indicators that will measure customer satisfaction. Other concerns include cost reduction and revenue enhancement.

Identifying Key Indicators

The assessment described in chapter 3 pinpoints the departments, services, and functions that are candidates for outsourcing. At the same time, interviews and questionnaires serve to identify the activities within a particular area that define good or superior performance in the opinion of the customer.

The following example should help to clarify the process. An ambulatory surgery center has historically developed and performed its own marketing. The marketing administrator was responsible for communication with the offices of those physicians who used the center's facilities and a secretary maintained the credentialing files. When the administrator resigned, the center's owners decided they needed to determine if there was a better way to market the center. Discussions with user physicians revealed that the previous communication system did not always provide their offices with needed information, there were delays and problems in the credentialing system that users felt were unnecessary, and there was no mechanism for discussion of issues and problems. The owners put together an operations team that further analyzed the situation and found that outsourcing the marketing function might prove cost-effective and also enhance the communication processes that users found inefficient.

Based on discussions with user physicians, office staff, and former patients, the team identified several indicators of performance that would be required of a vendor, including contacts with an office based on center utilization (i.e., practices that used the center the most would have the most frequent contact) and average time for a physician or practice to be credentialed. These criteria enabled the center to interview prospective providers of a liaison service and compare the guarantees of one service with another as well as with customer expectations. These indicators were incorporated into the outsourcing contract as well.

By reviewing the information obtained during the outsourcing assessment, the operations team can identify the activities that customers deem

FIGURE 4-1. Benchmarking Examples

Activity Being Evaluated	Benchmark	Source
Warehouse	Backorder rate	Other health care facilities Materials management organizations
Lease administration	Overhead cost per sq foot	Other health care facilities Real estate firms
Emergency medicine	X-rays per ER visit	Other health care facilities
Dietary services	Meal cost per patient day	Other health care facilities Hotel associations Dietitian groups
Housekeeping	Labor cost per sq foot	Other health care facilities Hotel associations National databases
Management of medical equipment	Average delivery time	Other health care facilities Hotel (compare to room service)
Sterilization services	Average turnaround time	Other health care facilities
Lab services	Average cost of lab test	Other health care facilities
Benefits administration	Hours of availability	Other health care facilities Other firms of similar size National HR groups
Equipment repair	Average repair time	Other health care facilities Professional organizations

(Continued on next page)

FIGURE 4-1. (Continued)

Activity Being Evaluated	Benchmark	Source
Facility management	Average cost per sq foot	Other health care facilities Architectural firms National organizations
Radiology asset management	Uptime on MRI unit	Other health care facilities Imaging centers
Laundry/linen service	Pounds per patient day	Other health care facilities Hotels
Respiratory management	Ventilator days per year	Other health care facilities Professional groups
Admissions office	Average wait time	Other health care facilities Airlines Any activity with a queue
Security service	FTE per sq foot	Other health care facilities Colleges and universities Airports

important. These can be compared to other organizations' experience to determine what steps must be taken to enhance the department, service, or function. A second important element of this process is that it can open lines of communication. In one hospital, for example, the sterilization department believed that a two-hour turnaround time on surgical trays was appropriate. However, interviews with operating room staff revealed that their expectation on turnaround time was under one hour. Before the outsourcing process could continue, this stumbling block had to be removed. Through meetings with both departments, a more realistic expectation of one and a half hours was agreed upon.

Choose Appropriate Benchmarks

After a list of performance indicators has been developed, it must be determined whether current performance is adequate. To do this, the organization must look to the experiences of other organizations. This is necessary because most customers use the services of other organizations and judge the performance of one against another. But perhaps more important, an organization must compare itself against its rivals in order to know where it stands.

Benchmarking has been a fairly common practice in a number of industries, and recently it has become more prevalent in health care. This is because health care organizations must continually improve their performance in light of the increased competition for patients. Benchmarking becomes a way to see where an organization stands today and where it must go in the future in order to compete successfully. The use of benchmarking in the outsourcing process ensures that the desired level of performance is communicated to potential vendors during the proposal process. In addition, the benchmarks become a yardstick to monitor the performance of the vendor over the life of the outsourcing contract.

Some health care organizations reach the benchmarking stage and then simply contact the facility down the street as a source of comparisons. However, this can be a mistake. Benchmarks should be acquired from a facility that performs an activity efficiently and effectively, leading to the best outcomes (such as cost reduction or patient satisfaction), and not from one that happens to be located in the neighborhood.

Another pitfall to avoid in choosing benchmarks is that of relying solely on customer satisfaction. Although it is true that the bottom line must be to improve customer satisfaction, customer feedback can be subjective and not representative of all the customers using that particular department, service, or function. Rather than assuming that any intervention will enhance satisfaction, the goal must be to benchmark only activities that will bring about such a result. For instance, having reading materials available in a waiting room might enhance customer satisfaction, but would not be a reliable indicator of customer satisfaction because taste varies and not every selection will please every customer.

Another pitfall in setting benchmarks is that of relying on customer expectations. For example, one hospital was developing benchmarks for the delivery of supplies requested by nursing units over the telephone.

Interviews with the nurse managers revealed that they desired a two-hour response time to telephone requests. The process was monitored, revealing that the actual response time was twenty minutes. In this case, the expectations of the customers were much lower than what existed. More important, had no external checks been done, the organization might have set the level of expectation for the outsourcing vendor at too low a threshold.

Identifying Types of Benchmark Sources.   The information needed to benchmark an activity may be found in a variety of sources. The key concept is to choose "the best of the best" when selecting one. The best of the best may be identified by the following:

- Conducting an on-line search to find organizations that are leaders in their areas
- Contacting associations such as the Public Relations Society of America to identify managers who are recognized by their peers or to locate organizations that have received industry recognition
- Searching health care trade publications to find organizations that have been profiled in the media

Two types of sources are health care and non-health care sources.

- *Health care sources:* Benchmark information can be obtained from a variety of other health care providers. Often a similar type of organization, which performs a similar activity, will serve as a source. Examples include hospitals, ambulatory surgery centers, outpatient radiology sites, and physician offices. Trade groups and professional groups may also prove helpful, such as the American Hospital Association, state hospital associations, or the Long Term Care Group. In addition, benchmarks can be purchased from a variety of commercial organizations. However, the purchase of benchmarks is usually reserved for select situations or to benchmark clinical outcomes.
- *Non-health care sources:* Some activities that are to be benchmarked resemble tasks performed in non-health care areas. For instance, dietary and cleaning activities cross industry lines and can be compared against the other industries. Often health care organizations may find it helpful to look at the cleaning of a hotel room when looking at cleaning patient rooms. Another example

is the delivery of items from central distribution in response to telephone requests; some facilities have found this comparable to the room service function and used it as a benchmark. The key to going outside of health care is to identify similar activities and to develop a complete understanding of what tasks make up the activities.

Contacting Sources of Benchmarks. When contacting a potential source of benchmarks, it is important to fully explain the benchmarking process. This should include a description of purpose and activity, how the facility was chosen, and how the information will be used. The information received from the other organization should be treated with confidentiality.

Sometimes the provider of the benchmarks may want information in return, in terms of either other benchmarks or the outcome of the outsourcing process. Therefore, the operations team should be prepared to share their findings with these outside managers. If the operations team is not forthcoming, future collaboration may be compromised.

Unlike other industries in which manufacturing processes and product ingredients are closely guarded, health care has relatively few trade secrets. Therefore, if simple guidelines are followed, such as those recommended by the Strategic Planning Institute and the American Productivity and Quality Center's Code of Conduct, obtaining the cooperation of other health care organizations should be fairly easy. See figure 4-2 for an example of a benchmarking code of conduct.

FIGURE 4-2. Benchmarking Code of Conduct

- Conduct yourself within legal bounds
- Exchange information
- Respect confidentiality
- Use the information only for the stated purpose
- Initiate contacts with individuals who have been identified through personal contact or through referrals from colleagues
- Obtain permission before referring others to a contact
- Be prepared for each contact with a list of questions and desired information
- Follow through on any commitments made to a benchmarking contact (e.g., did you promise to share results?)
- Treat information from others as they request

Using Benchmarks Effectively.   Benchmarks should be compared to internal functions. The two critical points at this juncture are the accuracy of the benchmarks and the parallels between internal and external functions. For example:

- *Benchmark accuracy:* Review data to ensure reliability. One surgery center obtained a benchmark on sterilization turn-around of 45 minutes per tray. Upon review, it was noted that the cycle time for the sterilizer itself was 40 minutes, leaving only five minutes to wash and pack the tray. This raised suspicions about the validity of the external benchmark.
- *Parallels between external and internal function:* One hospital benchmarked the activities performed in their print shop, with an eye toward outsourcing the department. When gathering information from other organizations, the operations team was faced with some comparability issues. The internal department was responsible for the maintenance of all copiers throughout the facility, forms were printed on a press as well as a high-speed copier, and the staff assisted department managers to develop needed forms. These services were not conducted by the departments of other organizations.

It is imperative that the tasks and factors that make up an activity are understood so that the comparison is accurate. An example of the effective use of benchmarks is presented in the following case study.

APPLYING BENCHMARKS AS PERFORMANCE INDICATORS: A CASE STUDY

An organization that provides subacute care has determined that benefits administration is not an area of critical importance to its success. In addition, recent meetings with employees revealed a fairly high level of dissatisfaction with current services. The assessment phase (outlined in chapter 3) was completed and revealed the following key indicators of performance:

- Written material available to employees at all five of the organization's sites (Currently these materials had to be picked up at the organization's corporate headquarters.)

- Representatives familiar with various benefits available to answer questions to staff on all shifts (Benefits staff were available 9 A.M. to 5 P.M., Monday through Friday.)
- Information about changes to current benefits and about new ones communicated in a timely fashion (Informational pamphlets were distributed quarterly to staff.)

In reviewing these key indicators, the operations team determined it would be cost-prohibitive to attempt such activities internally. However, before contacting outside vendors, the organization wanted to know how it stacked up against other organizations. Three sources were identified: a local hospital that had similar-sized staff but was located at only one site, a long-term care organization with three sites, and a (nonunion) manufacturing firm with six sites. The results of calls to these provided the following information:

- Organizations with multiple sites provided informational brochures at each location.
- Organizations with staff on multiple shifts did not routinely provide benefits staff availability on the evening or night shift. (One did provide early morning [7 A.M.] access one day a month.)
- Each of the organizations included new or changed benefit information in the monthly employee newsletter.

The operations team first investigated the feasibility of an employee newsletter. Although this had been discussed in the past, no action had ever been taken. The operations team was able to launch the newsletter, which included a human resource/benefits section.

The other indicators of performance were planned for outsourcing and incorporated into a request for proposal. (See chapter 7.) At a minimum, the operations team expected to identify firms that would provide 24-hour access through a toll-free telephone center and a mechanism to provide written material on a regular basis at each site.

CONCLUSION

Benchmarking allows an organization to evaluate internal performance against outside standards of excellence. Properly executed, the benchmarking procedure enables the organization to identify internal weaknesses and provide potential remedies. Benchmarking can also assist the outsourcing team in setting standards for vendors and in preparing requests for proposals.

Once a clear picture of activities is obtained and a list of potential outsourcing candidates developed, the organization can move to the next step. To complete the analysis, the health care organization must project revenue and expenses into the future for both internal and out-sourced management of the department, service, or function. This is covered in the next chapter.

5

Developing Baseline Projections

The next step in the outsourcing process is to project the required volume of a service or activity. This is necessary to properly size the contract (discussed in chapter 8). Obviously, the volume or quantity of service will not remain constant over the next three to five years, so a projection must be made in order to ensure that the service levels match the demand the health care organization expects to have in the future. Detailed information on projections of demand, expenses, and revenues is beyond the scope of this book. Rather, the intention here is to present the concepts and relate them to the outsourcing process. However, this in no way minimizes the need to calculate these numbers to accurately assess the proposals submitted by outsourcing vendors.

This chapter examines the components involved in making projections of future service demands and in making financial projections for comparison against outsourcing proposal costs. It also presents a case study showing how a health care facility projected potential demand for a cardiac service when trying to decide whether to offer the service in-house or to outsource it.

BENEFITS OF DETERMINING FUTURE NEEDS

The operations team can accurately determine the costs of an outsourcing contract over its life. The results of this process can be used to prepare and/or revise an organization's budget and long-range plan or it can provide a basis for financing capital projects. Because of the detailed nature of these projections, the outcome will provide an accurate picture of an organization's current status and a prudent estimate of its potential. By analyzing requirements for the future, the team will begin to understand how their decision will affect the organization for years to come. Other benefits include the timing of related activities, anticipating need for additional resources, and preparing the ground for ongoing monitoring.

DEMAND PROJECTIONS

A demand projection consists of calculations that reveal the volume of services that a population, organization, or department will be required to provide to its customers. After the demand level is estimated, financial projections can be calculated to show the income and/or expense related to the activity. The results of the financial projections will be the basis of comparison for the various outsourcing proposals.

Demand projections must be made in terms of both nonclinical and clinical activities. These are discussed in the following subsections.

Nonclinical Activities

In estimating the demand for nonclinical activities, it is usually appropriate to use historical information, which can be tied to some future level of service or volume indicator to project the demand. For instance, the demand placed on a laundry department can be estimated using the historical pounds of linen per patient day. Future demand is simply a matter of applying the ratio to projected patient days. This simple formula can be applied in a variety of situations, provided that an appropriate volume indicator is available.

Difficulties may arise when the volume indicator is unavailable or if some organizational change alters the demand pattern. For instance, one surgical center had to consider the impact that universal precautions would have on its impervious surgical gown supply when developing its laundry contract. The administrator's best guess was an increase of 4 gowns per day, or 20 additional per week. While this might sound insignificant to a multihospital system, it can adversely affect a freestanding center with two operating rooms.

Clinical Activities

To estimate the demand for clinical services, projections must be made for inpatient and/or outpatient services. Two key tools in predicating the level of service are use rates and market share. In calculating these measurements, it is advisable to use figures for at least the past two or three years to eliminate any unusual fluctuations that may have occurred because of one-time events.

Determining Use Rates.   Use rates represent the relationship between population data and demand data for either the particular health care institution or all organizations of a similar nature (for example, all long-term care facilities). The formula for determining use rate is:

Use rate = total admissions or visits for target organizations
$$\frac{\text{in the service area}}{\text{total population of the service area}}$$

where service area is defined as the geographic region in which most of the health care organization's services are delivered. This can vary depending on the type and location of the organization. For instance, the service area of an inner-city physician practice may be limited to two or three zip codes, while that of a rural practice may be an entire county. Definition of the service area dramatically affects use rates by shrinking or expanding the number of potential users of a service.

Moreover, when calculating use rates, it may be necessary to calculate separate rates for specific population groups. For instance, in projecting the use for MRI services, there may be a difference in rate between those individuals under age 65 and those over. This can have an impact on demand.

Use rates tend to remain fairly constant over time. However, certain factors can affect the rate, such as changes in reimbursement or government regulations. The operations team must be aware of potential trends that could alter future use. For example, the use rate for inpatient cardiac stays may decrease with the advent of nonsurgical interventions.

Calculating Market Share.   The proportion of services provided by an organization versus total services delivered in the organization's service area defines a specific health care provider's market share. This is calculated as follows:

$$\text{Market share} = \frac{\text{service area admissions, visits, or volume for the health care provider}}{\text{total service area admissions, visits, or volume}}$$

This calculation reveals what portion of volume in the service area is being captured by the specific health care entity. For instance, a facility that is trying to decide whether to add a women's center would need to know what percentage of women's services are presently being captured. This can reveal whether a competitor has "sewn up the market" or whether opportunities in fact exist. In addition, it will paint a picture of how well the organization has been able to attract women to the facility without an organized program.

In projecting market share, factors that may affect future share should be considered, such as internal plans to expand or contract related services or a competitor's plan. The operations team must gather as much information as possible on these issues in order to accurately project the needed level of service.

Projecting Demand for Service.   After use rates and market share have been calculated, the operations team can project future demand. Most activities, whether clinical or supportive, will not remain flat. Volume may increase because of increased utilization, changes in technology, or other factors. Likewise, volume may decrease as a result of shifts in population or new technologies. Moreover, specific factors may be unique to a particular organization. For instance, if an assisted living facility opens in a rural area, demand for home health services may decline as individuals relocate to the facility.

Another possibility is that some services may show an increase if complementary services are expanded. For instance, one hospital found that its emergency room visits were decreasing because of lack of critical care beds. A planned expansion of the intensive care unit was projected to increase ER visits by 25 percent. This factor had to be considered when the facility was evaluating the possibility of outsourcing the management of the ER.

A number of factors must be considered when projecting demand for inpatient services. These include the following:

- Service area (typically defined as those zip codes or census tracts that provide more than 80 percent of historical admissions)

- Current and projected population data
- Competition
- Use rates
- Market share
- Market forces such as payer mix and managed care penetration
- Medical staff stability, age, and allegiance and practice ownership
- Current and future services

Projecting Volume of Service.   One other factor to consider is the volume of service, which depends on the number of inpatients and outpatients treated. For example, utilization of transcription services depends on volume of inpatient admissions and outpatient visits for ancillary services. Utilization of physical therapy, laboratory, and radiology will vary depending on emergency visits, inpatient admissions, clinic visits, and outpatient referrals. The relationship between inpatient services and outpatient services will differ depending on the area being examined. That is, the percent of outpatient volume in the lab to total outpatient visits may be significantly different than that of radiology.

The volume demand may be estimated based on the relationship between the volume of the department and overall hospital volume. These relationships can be calculated with data that are readily available. For example, projecting the volume for the dietary department would involve the following calculation:

$$\text{Patient meals} = \frac{\text{historical patient meals for 1 year}}{\text{total patient days for 1 year}} \times \text{projected patient days}$$

This calculation does not consider outpatient visits because the dietary department does not provide meals to outpatients. For departments with an outpatient component, an additional calculation would account for outpatient volume, as shown below:

$$\text{Radiology exams} = \frac{\text{inpatient radiology exams}}{\text{total admissions}} \times \text{projected admissions} +$$
$$\frac{\text{outpatient radiology exams}}{\text{total outpatient visits}} \times \text{projected outpatient visits}$$

FINANCIAL PROJECTIONS

After use rates, market share, demand, and volume are projected, this information can be used to generate projected financial statements. The operations team will need to understand what the internal costs are in order to compare the outsourcing proposal costs.

The need to project revenue, expenses, or both is dependent on the structure of the outsourcing agreement. One case is the management agreement, where the outsourcing vendor will assume complete responsibility for staffing, supplies, management, and other expenses. The operations team will need projections of internal expenses only, since revenue will not be affected. Another situation exists when the outsourcing vendor also assumes responsibility for billing and collections. In this case, the operations team must have information on projected revenue in order to evaluate what will be the terms of the agreement.

The department's expenses and revenues, as projected by the health care organization, should be used to compare the proposed costs under the vendor proposal. The internal and external projections must be assessed to ensure that they contain the same elements.

Following are many of the internal costs that must be considered when making financial projections:

- Salaries
- Fringe benefits
- Professional fees
- Insurance
- Maintenance contracts
- Supplies
- Equipment
- Transition expense

These are discussed in the following subsections.

Salaries

Expenses associated with the staff of a department should be projected, either by position or in total. Projected staffing would be adjusted based on changes in projected volume, changes in services, and any known or planned changes in positions. To calculate salaries, multiply average salary by full-time-equivalent employees. Salaries should be adjusted for potential increase in volume as well as planned salary increases.

In projecting salary expenses, current conditions and expected trends in the labor pool must be considered. While there may currently be an excess of qualified candidates, the situation may change drastically over the next three to five years. The reasons may include changes in job seekers' tastes, compensation opportunities, and expansion of employment opportunities in other fields. Conversely, shortages today may correct themselves in the long run as individuals are drawn into the field. The size of the labor pool may change salary structures and benefits; it may even necessitate additional expenditures on recruitment fees, relocation expenses, and advertising expenses. The operations team must consider these factors in projecting future costs.

Fringe Benefits

Fringe benefits are noncash compensation items such as health insurance, life insurance, disability insurance, and pension plan payments. Generally, fringe benefits are projected based on a percentage of base salary. This can be based on the historical percentage of benefits to total payroll. Many health care organizations do not charge benefits directly to the department. Others only charge a portion of the benefit expenses to individual areas. Although an individual department manager may not see these expenses, it is important to include them in the projection so that an accurate picture of expenses can be developed.

Professional Fees

Professional fees are the expenses associated with payments to external entities for services rendered internally. While these are typically monies paid to physicians, there are other expenditures that may be classified as professional fees; for instance, fees paid to an advertising agency, employment search firms, and information systems support. These fees should be projected in the same manner as they are currently incurred. For instance, if the fee is currently a fixed monthly fee, it

should be projected as a fixed monthly fee, perhaps adjusted for inflation. If there are multiple professional fees involved, they should be separated and projected separately.

Insurance

Outsourcing agreements may have no effect on an organization's insurance needs. In such cases, there would be no need to project the
expense. However, some arrangements allow for a shift in liability to the
outsource provider, in which case the organization may be able to
decrease the amount of insurance carried. This will decrease the projected cost of insurance and should be included in the analysis.

Maintenance Contracts

Some outsourcing agreements cover new and existing equipment for
which a maintenance contract may be in place. If the outsourcing vendor will assume responsibility for maintenance and repair, the health
care facility will have no reason to keep the maintenance contract. In
such cases, the decreased expense projection should be included in the
financial analysis. A second consideration is the age and condition of
current equipment. Increases in volume will place additional strain on
older equipment, potentially causing more breakdowns and shorter
operating life. In addition, if the outsourcing proposal calls for the vendor to provide newer technology, maintenance contracts may become
unnecessary through the initial years of ownership. All such factors
must be considered when assessing the financial implications of an outsourcing contract.

Supplies

Supplies to be used in the performance of the activity being considered
for outsourcing must be included in the financial analysis. Typically,
these costs are projected based on a cost-per-volume indicator. For
instance, one facility wanted to project the cost of disposable respiratory
supplies. Using historical rates ($3.11 per patient day) and projected

volumes (164,871 patient days), they were able to project these supplies at over $500,000 annually. This was compared with the cost quoted in outsourcing proposals dealing with management of the respiratory therapy department.

Equipment

Some departments or functions are heavily dependent on equipment. Examples include laboratory, radiology, sterilization, and dietary. Equipment may or may not be included in outsourcing proposals. If it is included, the operations team must take into consideration the effect that transfer of responsibility will have on internal expenses. In such cases, the operations team will need information regarding the increase or decrease and any change in cash payments.

Transition Expense

One of the final issues that must be considered is the cost that may be associated with transition to the outsourcing vendor. Many times, duplicate services will be running while the responsibilities are handed over to the vendor; for example, implementation of accounting software when outsourcing outpatient billing. While this will not last long, it may be long enough to warrant analysis of associated expenses.

PROJECTING DEMAND FOR CARDIAC SERVICES: A CASE STUDY

A health care organization is considering the addition of cardiac catheterization services. Ultimately, there is the choice of providing the program internally or outsourcing it to one of several vendors that will develop and manage the service. Before proceeding, the organization must determine what the demand for such services might be based on use rates and market share. As an example, three-year calculations of historical use rates and market share for an organization's cardiac services are shown in figure 5-1.

**FIGURE 5-1. Historical Use Rate and Market Share
             for Cardiac Services**

Historical Use Rate

Year 1 = $\dfrac{24{,}287 \text{ total service area admissions}}{928{,}180 \text{ total population}}$ × 1,000 = 26.2 admissions/1,000

Year 2 = $\dfrac{24{,}162 \text{ total service area admissions}}{928{,}180 \text{ total population}}$ × 1,000 = 26.0 admissions/1,000

Year 3 = $\dfrac{25{,}531 \text{ total service area admissions}}{928{,}180 \text{ total population}}$ × 1,000 = 27.5 admissions/1,000

3-year average = 26.6 admissions/1,000

Historical Market Share

Year 1 = $\dfrac{2{,}638 \text{ hospital-specific cardiac admissions}}{24{,}287 \text{ service area cardiac admissions}}$ = 10.9%

Year 2 = $\dfrac{2{,}846 \text{ hospital-specific cardiac admissions}}{24{,}162 \text{ service area cardiac admissions}}$ = 11.8%

Year 3 = $\dfrac{2{,}795 \text{ hospital-specific cardiac admissions}}{25{,}531 \text{ service area cardiac admissions}}$ = 10.9%

3-year average = 11.1%

These numbers are then used to project the demand for cardiac services. Likewise, the organization will use the projected cardiac admissions to project increases in ancillary and support services. For instance, if cardiac admissions are projected to increase by 380 patients due to the addition of the cardiac cath lab, radiology will perform 756 additional exams using a historical inpatient rate of 1.99 procedures per inpatient discharge. These additional exams, along with additional volume in other departments, must be factored into the total projected volume for the institution.

CONCLUSION

Developing projections is more than just identifying current trends. It is considering all factors that may change the volume of services delivered by the health care organization and projecting their effect on expense and revenue. Then the results of this process can be compared to outsourcing proposals to determine whether outsourcing will have a positive or negative financial impact. Long-range plans must be considered so that an organization's requirements over the life of an outsourcing contract can be fully appreciated.

Developing projections allows a health care institution to properly size requirements for staff and services. This will be used to write both the request for proposals (chapter 7) and the final contract (chapter 8). In addition, inclusion of realistic projections in the RFP allows vendors to respond in a comprehensive fashion. This should afford a health care organization a better opportunity in selecting a vendor to perform the outsourced service.

6

Identifying Potential Partners

Having identified candidates for outsourcing, projected demand for these services in the future, and estimated the full cost associated with the services, departments, or functions to be outsourced, it is time to identify the vendors who have the expertise and capabilities to provide the highest-quality services in a cost-effective manner. However, before requesting proposals from potential vendors, health care organizations should develop a strategy for evaluating them.

This chapter presents a step-by-step method for evaluating and selecting potential vendors and explores the advantages and disadvantages of three different outsourcing arrangements.

TYPES OF OUTSOURCING ARRANGEMENTS

To identify potential partners, the team should plot out a methodological approach that will produce the most thoughtful and thorough evaluation of each vendor's strengths and weaknesses. Once a vendor is chosen, all parties concerned in the outsourcing arrangement will understand why this vendor was selected as the best qualified to undertake the project.

The first step in selecting a vendor is to determine the most appropriate structure for the outsourcing arrangement. Using one or many vendors is a choice that depends on the health care system's culture, the vendors, and the specific job at hand. The health care organization may use multiple vendors, an umbrella vendor, or a group purchasing organization

(GPO). Each of these arrangements is discussed below, along with its advantages and disadvantages.

Multiple Vendors

In some cases, organizations choose many vendors, believing each will provide the highest level of service in its area of expertise. There is some sense to this. It may be easier to imagine that a vendor with experience in a particular area will provide superior service in its area of expertise than to believe that one firm can have expertise in a number of unrelated areas.

Advantages of Multiple Vendors.   Using multiple vendors can provide several advantages. First, contracting with various companies creates a competitive environment. Health care organizations have found that this affords them added control over vendors, as individual companies attempt to "outdo" the other firms, thus avoiding any tendency to become complacent. Second, multiple competitors offer a safety net against problems, such as interruptions in service due to work stoppage resulting from contract disputes. The mere fact that there are other companies involved with a health care system increases its ability to bargain—one vendor cannot exert undue influence on the smooth operation of your organization. And third, using multiple vendors affords access to a large pool of talented individuals who can provide added expertise to daily operations.

Disadvantages of Multiple Vendors.   On the negative side, using multiple vendors involves writing more contracts. This translates into additional negotiations, meetings, and monitoring efforts, which may counterbalance the benefits of using multiple vendors. The involvement of additional external staff may also result in a fragmented flow of information. Although this can be overcome, it becomes more difficult as more companies are brought into the picture. In addition, multiple vendors introduce multiple organizational cultures into a health care system, because they are required to mesh not only with your hospital staff, but also with employees from other organizations.

Umbrella Vendors

Some organizations favor umbrella vendors: one source providing a number of unrelated services. Although small companies may be unable to develop expertise in many areas, large national firms have been able to offer expertise in several departments or functions, typically support areas. For example, an umbrella vendor might offer dietary services, warehouse and distribution management, housekeeping, and facilities management.

Advantages of Umbrella Vendors.   Umbrella vendors provide economies of scale that can result in lower costs. If supplies and/or equipment are included in the outsourcing agreement, the umbrella vendor may be able to provide them at a much lower cost than the hospital can obtain on its own. The same would hold for the staff provided by the vendor. The savings generated can benefit the health care organization greatly.

Umbrella vendors also offer economies of scope. When companies either produce multiple products or perform a service at many locations, the learning curve for workers decreases. Although there may be subtle differences in performance expectations at various sites, they know the basic process and can "hit the ground running." For instance, an employee of a facilities management firm can use internal policies and procedures as well as experience at another client site to make the transition to a new client site easier and quicker.

Umbrella vendors also decrease the administrative burden on the health care system. Rather than meeting with five vendors to discuss five departments, a hospital manager can meet with one representative to discuss all five areas. Dealing with one vendor thus streamlines the process and improves communication. Umbrella vendors offer other advantages including tremendous resources and ability to recruit staff.

Disadvantages of Umbrella Vendors.   On the downside, the level of expertise that an umbrella vendor has in any specific area may never reach the level that one specialized company immersed in an activity can possess. For instance, a vendor that exclusively provides management of a sub-acute unit will develop expertise in the applicable regulations and billing procedures. This expertise may be much less developed in a vendor that provides management of several types of alternate-care facilities.

In addition, health care organizations should be wary of becoming dependent on one umbrella vendor. As more departments and functions are shifted to one vendor, the organization may begin to rely on that vendor exclusively. Should the vendor fail, the organization may suffer.

Group Purchasing Organizations

A GPO is an association of a number of independent entities that band together in order to achieve a balance of power in contract negotiations. Some GPOs have begun offering outsourcing contracts to their members. These canned products may or may not meet the needs of a specific organization.

Advantages of Group Purchasing Organizations.   Some GPO contracts are extremely beneficial, offering significant savings to member institutions, especially for activities and programs that are standardized in all institutions and require no customization. Examples of these are rare, but may include management of the parking garage or the coffee shop.

Disadvantages of Group Purchasing Organizations.   Other contracts are somewhat problematic because the same program is offered to all members. If programs are not customized to address specific issues of an organization, there is no way to quantify savings attributable to the GPO. Unless these issues are adequately addressed, the GPO offerings may not hold any advantages over what an organization can negotiate for itself.

FACTORS INFLUENCING VENDOR SELECTION

The type of outsourcing arrangement to use can and should be determined before developing a request for proposal (discussed in chapter 7). This decision depends on a number of variables, including:

- Organizational culture
- Type of vendor

- Impact on patient care
- Complexity of the activity

Organizational Culture

It is important that the operations team develop a philosophy regarding the use of multiple or umbrella vendors or a GPO before seeking vendors to bid on a project. The selection is a function of the health care organization's culture. For example, an organization's past experiences with outsourcing are likely to color its future decisions. Thus, it may be important to research a health care system's history of using contract services, which may provide insight into the arrangement that will be the most productive.

Type of Vendor

In some cases, the health care organization's current vendors may offer the service or function being considered for outsourcing. If the organization has a solid relationship with its current vendor, there may be no reason to search for a new one. However, often it may be wise to seek the input of several vendors in an effort to determine which ones offer the best-quality product in a cost-effective manner. In such a case, the operations team should develop a database of potential vendors. (See figure 6-1).

Certainly, one aspect of identifying qualified potential vendors is deciding on the type of vendor sought. Vendors under consideration for an outsourcing contract may include support vendors, clinical vendors, business vendors, or new entrants into vending for the health care industry.

Support Vendors.   Support vendors provide auxiliary services such as housekeeping, dietary, plant maintenance, facilities management, warehouse management, distribution, sterilization, transportation, linen/laundry, print shop, telecommunications, clinical engineering, medical records, transcription, and equipment service. GPOs, health care societies, professional magazines and journals related to the area to be outsourced, and manufacturer/seller groups may serve as resources in identifying potential support vendors. Because large national "umbrella" vendors often provide support services, determine if any vendors currently providing services to the health care system also provide other services that are not currently being used.

FIGURE 6-1. Developing a Database of Vendors

A database of vendors should include:

- Name, address, and telephone numbers of potential company
- Year established
- Year in which the company began to offer the particular activity you seek
- Other services offered
- Number of contracts or clients the company currently has
- Number of health care organizations served
- Historical annual sales or revenues for three to five years
- Public or private status
- Geographical spread of clients
- Recent publicity
- Financial status
- Names, addresses, and phone numbers of satisfied clients (preferably in the health care industry)

Clinical Vendors. Clinical vendors often specialize in a particular specialty, such as emergency room management, pharmacy, wound care, subacute unit management, quality assurance, bone densitometry, radiology film interpretation, physical therapy, radiation therapy, clinical laboratory, employee health, respiratory therapy, and home care. The best sources for potential clinical vendors are professional organizations that publish journal articles on the programs provided by various vendors and advertisers (for example, the American Association for Clinical Chemistry or the American College of Clinical Pharmacy).

Another resource for information on clinical vendors might be the manufacturer of equipment used in the department being considered for outsourcing. For instance, if outsourcing respiratory therapy is under consideration, ventilator manufacturers may be a good source for a vendor reference; for radiology-related services, radiology equipment manufacturers may offer suggestions for potential vendors. Manufacturers may offer the service themselves or may be aware of potential vendors through their experiences with other facilities.

Business Vendors. Health care systems may consider outsourcing business functions, including cashier, accounts receivable, accounts payable, real estate management, contract management, legal services, and lock box services. To identify potential providers, the organization might consult business journals and firms that provide auditing services for recommendations.

New Health Care Vendors.   Normally, a health care organization would not seek out firms that traditionally provided services to another industry but are expanding to include the health care industry. However, these firms may offer value-added services if the activity under consideration for outsourcing is specialized and directly related to the distinctive competency of the vendor. For instance, a vendor with experience in retail warehousing or distribution may be a good candidate for medical/surgical supply management.

Impact on Patient Care

Another factor to consider is the impact that a vendor may have on care, especially if the outsourced service is one that is extremely visible to the patient population. A novice vendor may compromise quality of care. If there has been negative publicity about the potential vendor, it may have a negative impact on the hospital's credibility. If the service/activity to be outsourced is not involved in direct patient care, the impact will be low and there is less concern as to your choice of vendors.

Complexity of the Activity

Uncomplicated tasks that cross organizational lines, such as housekeeping or grounds maintenance, can be completed effectively and efficiently by many companies. Therefore, these functions could be outsourced with confidence to either one or many firms. On the other hand, complex tasks, such as billing or radiation therapy, require a much higher degree of skill and knowledge. These tasks should be outsourced to a highly specialized firm whose only focus is the target activity.

METHOD FOR CHOOSING A VENDOR

The actual process of selecting a vendor for outsourcing a function, service, or department involves two steps: doing preliminary research and then evaluating the vendor based on the information obtained through that research.

Preliminary Research

Before requesting proposals, the operations team should request pre-bidding information to confirm that potential suppliers can meet the objectives of the health care organization and that the vendor is capable of delivering the service in an efficient, dependable, timely fashion. This information may streamline the process by eliminating some firms from consideration.

In addition, the team might seek information on vendors from the Internet; company Web pages, on-line news media sources, and government sites all may contain useful information. However, it is important to remember that the information available from a company's Web site has been developed for marketing purposes and may not provide the entire story. Business publications or industry analyses can provide more valuable background information on potential vendors. Another source of information might be health care trade groups such as the American Hospital Association (AHA), the Medical Group Management Association (MGMA), or the American Healthcare Association (AHCA).

Besides seeking out information about the vendor on the Internet or through publications, members of the organization's operations team might visit the potential vendor's facility, especially those that may have a systemwide impact on an organization, such as one involving telecommunications or computer systems. The logistics of providing a tour of a facility may be prohibitive, however, especially for larger corporations, and the team members may have to rely on other sources, including satisfied client references provided by the potential vendor.

Evaluating Vendors

There are two approaches to consider when evaluating vendors: the participatory approach and the administrative or management approach.

Participatory Approach.   The participatory approach is an excellent approach to use when considering a function that affects several departments, such as transportation, clinical engineering, and lock box management. By forming a vendor selection team composed of members from each department involved, all departments affected by the outsourcing can be included in the evaluation process. Membership on this team should be limited to five to seven people; a larger team will be less efficient.

Because each department has particular concerns that could pose problems to a vendor's efficient operation, identifying these concerns up front allows the potential vendor to address each item specifically. Thus, the team will be better able to assess the vendor's ability to produce a satisfactory outcome for the outsourced department. For example, when considering clinical engineering for outsourcing, the affected departments will have different concerns: central sterilization is concerned by the turnaround time on repairs of movable equipment, administration is concerned with expenditures for a parts inventory, and quality assurance is concerned about compliance with regulatory standards. A representative of each area should participate on the vendor selection team either directly or through surveys, so that concerns regarding time, expense, and quality control can each be addressed by the vendor.

Administrative or Management Approach.   An administrative or management approach should be reserved for sensitive situations or those involving union contracts. For example, if an activity earmarked for outsourcing is currently performed under a collective bargaining agreement, it would be appropriate to use an administrative approach in evaluating vendors.

Other situations calling for an administrative or management approach include the outsourcing of areas where an entire department may be eliminated, where there is physician involvement, or where the interests of the organization are best served by limiting the number of individuals involved in the process. In this approach, members of the vendor selection team should include only administrative staff. However, because there may be a need for sensitive information, key department heads such as human resources and finance should also be considered for inclusion. By paying attention to the details and proceeding in a methodical fashion, the vendor selection team can provide an important link in the successful implementation of an outsourcing agreement—one that could have made a big difference for the hospital cited in the following case study.

OUTSOURCING A CLINICAL SERVICE: A CASE STUDY

The president of a suburban hospital was informed by the facility's only vascular surgeon that he had entered into an agreement with another institution and would be leaving in three months. In addition, the two technicians who worked in the vascular department had accepted positions at the other facility. This left a void, and although this was not a large service for the institution, there were several contracts that required the hospital to provide vascular surgery.

The president identified two possible options: recruiting a vascular surgeon and staff or outsourcing the department to a qualified vendor. Although the president believed he would maintain more control if he were to recruit a surgeon, he knew this option would be costly. In addition, recruitment might take a significant amount of time, and he only had three months. A nearby medical center president, who thought her staff could provide the desired level of service in a cost-effective manner, then approached the president. Specifically, she offered twenty-four-hour coverage by a board-qualified vascular surgeon, certified vascular technicians, and management of the area. After discussing this proposal with the medical staff, the president was confident that this was the best choice and proceeded to sign an agreement with the teaching facility to start the program on April 1.

On March 25, the president was made aware of a potential problem. The staff of his institution was not covered by any collective bargaining agreements. However, the teaching facility was fully unionized, including the technicians who were to provide vascular service. The two hospital presidents worked out an arrangement whereby the teaching facility provided vascular surgeon coverage, while the hospital was responsible for the technicians. To meet the immediate needs of the area, the president authorized staffing from a temporary agency. Recruitment activities were initiated by human resources to fill the positions on a long-term basis. These actions allowed the provision of vascular services to continue uninterrupted.

Three months into the contract, the vascular surgeons informed the president that the equipment in the vascular lab was unacceptable and would need replacement. The cost of new equipment was estimated at approximately $250,000. Though there was no provision for this capital, the president believed he had to purchase the machinery or risk losing vascular surgeon coverage.

Discussion

While the vascular surgeon and staff clearly left the facility in the lurch, there was no reason to believe that the teaching facility's offer was the best approach. First, there does not appear to have been an adequate investigation before this offer was accepted. Second, because the agreement was hammered out at high levels of authority, attention to detail was lost. Allowing lower levels of staff to be involved might have prevented some serious oversights, such as those that occurred here. Finally, since there was no request for proposal (RFP), the institution had no way to determine what the future needs of the area would be. These considerations would be especially important in a smaller institution where capital funds are limited.

Recommendations

A number of recommendations might be drawn from this scenario, including:

- Whenever a situation such as this one becomes known, a small group of involved individuals should be brought together to develop a short list of requirements/performance criteria for the department affected.
- The RFP developed by this team should clearly state the implementation date and list departmental requirements. The RFP should also be structured with a very short response time.
- All potential vendors should be informed that the performance criteria would be limited for the first six months, but would expand as the vendor becomes more familiar with the needs of the institution.
- A description (make and model) of current equipment should be included in the RFP, and the vendor should be asked to review this information and advise if changes appear necessary. In addition, the vendor should obtain price quotes for any purchases deemed necessary and identify who will be responsible for such purchases.
- A firm date should be set for when a decision must be made.

CONCLUSION

By applying a methodical approach to the process of selecting vendors, a health care system will be able to direct the RFP to qualified firms. Whether to use an umbrella vendor, many vendors, or a GPO is dependent on the specific requirements of each institution. However, deciding which approach to take is important, because it shapes the future activity required to outsource a particular service or activity.

7

Preparing a Request for Proposal

With the groundwork laid for outsourcing a service, department, or function and potential vendors identified, the health care organization now must turn its attention to preparing a request for proposal (RFP). An RFP documents the organization's requirements for the products or services it wishes to purchase. In many business settings, RFPs are difficult to write because the task of summarizing and detailing a project and its requirements may be pressured by the need to expedite the solution to an outstanding problem.

The challenge to writing an RFP is in refining the request to secure the best possible outcome. As business documents, RFPs have many standard items, such as requirements for references and project management proposals. Nonetheless, customizing an RFP to meet the health care organization's specific outsourcing needs enhances the likelihood of contracting the most qualified vendor and sends the message to bidders that the organization demands a thorough and carefully constructed proposal.

This chapter discusses methods for creating a successful RFP. These include choosing an author, establishing goals, writing and issuing the request, and evaluating proposals.

CHOOSING AN RFP AUTHOR

Preparations for writing the RFP first involve gathering all relevant information and then choosing an author to consolidate it into one document. The RFP must be written so that vendors can respond in objective terms.

Selecting an Internal Author

The operations team will select an RFP director, who will act as the principal author of the document and coordinate the development of sections of the document that he or she does not write. Typically, this individual is either the head of the department most directly affected by the outsourcing or a senior administrator. In the case of a busy, overburdened RFP director, a deputy should be named by management to work as the document writer and to act as a chief assistant to the RFP director. The purchasing manager, who generally has experience in developing such documents, might be a good candidate for this position.

Retaining an Outside Author

In outsourcing areas involving advanced technology or rapidly changing products and services, such as information technology, it may be advantageous to obtain the assistance of an outside consultant in developing an appropriate proposal. However, some health care organizations ultimately may want the winning bidder of a technology-intensive project to act as the advising consultant. In these instances, the RFP is a "solutions" proposal. In other words, the organization describes its current circumstances and performance goals and invites vendors to provide solutions. The "complete" proposal written with the help of a consultant differs from the solutions proposal. In a complete proposal, the health care organization specifies its needs for items such as hardware, software, and employee training and invites vendors to bid accordingly. The operations team must decide which type of RFP to create; the decision usually takes time as the team determines if in-house expertise is sufficient to write a complete proposal.

Retaining an outside consultant also may be considered for situations in which use of in-house resources creates a drain on current operations. For instance, if only one or two staff members are in a department, their extensive involvement in the operations team may be unrealistic.

ESTABLISHING RFP GOALS

In addition to the explicit mission of the operations team to establish goals for outsourcing, prepare an RFP, and select a provider of services or goods, an unspoken mission is to build consensus about the outsourcing project. Consensus building is especially important to alleviate interdepartmental rivalries and territorial disputes. Establishing goals for the RFP process may be the first opportunity to build a consensus about sensitive issues among the health care organization's staff and departments.

The operations team should consider the number of proposals that will receive in-depth review, determine the information required by potential vendors, and establish the basis on which the organization will compare vendors. If the RFP is complex, lengthy, and technically detailed, an evaluation scale may be used to help determine which proposal best meets the organization's needs. A point system is most common and practical, with a greater number of points assigned to those components of the outsourcing agreement identified as most important. This is described later in the chapter in the sample RFP scoring system.

WRITING A REQUEST FOR PROPOSAL

RFPs take many forms and ultimately reflect the culture of the institutions that generate them. A number of trade associations, professional organizations, and business publishing houses make standardized RFPs available. For instance, the Computer Systems Laboratory of the National Institute of Standards and Technology has developed a model RFP for open computer systems.[1] Standardized RFPs provide writers with a starting point, which is especially helpful for preparing complex documents that may be daunting in the early stages of development. However, because the procurement of services or products is a highly individualized process, model RFPs should not be used verbatim. A boilerplate request will produce boilerplate proposals. A customized request will produce superior proposals. As a general rule, the more technical a service or product, the more customized the RFP should be.

Because an RFP is essentially the first stage in the process of signing a contract, the time and money spent by a health care organization in preparing it will pay dividends later when the project proceeds smoothly, with a lesser likelihood of change orders and related cost increases. Details omitted in the RFP are likely to remain undiscovered until the process of providing a service is well under way.

Customizing an RFP can take many forms. Most likely, the customization will take the form of nuts-and-bolts issues related to the bid:

the detailed breakdown of costs, schedules, functional requirements, and responsibilities. However, as varied as RFPs may be, a typical document contains certain standard items, including:

- Executive summary
- Instructions to bidders
- Qualifications
- Project management and staffing
- Functional requirements
- Evaluation criteria
- Glossary of terms
- Description of vendors
- References
- Fees and costs
- Appendices

Many health care systems distribute all or part of their RFPs on computer disks. This eliminates the need for data entry when the proposals are returned and reduces the demand for paper. However, in providing vendors with the disk, it should be clearly stated that vendors cannot change the wording of the request, but are expected only to fill in the requested information.

Executive Summary

The executive summary presents an overview of the scope and priorities of the project. This overview should include the business issues that drive the decision to outsource and an outline of the technologies or services that will provide the solution. Vendors should receive the message that the proposed outsourcing project is a well-thought-out business proposal and has the potential for a long-term relationship. A well-written executive summary sets the tone for the remaining sections of the RFP and will affect the vendors' response to it. For their part, most vendors want to spend as little time as possible in writing proposals as a hedge against not receiving the business. An RFP that immediately commands attention and respect is more likely to inspire thoughtful solutions from vendors.

Instructions to Bidders

The instructions to bidders section should outline the procedures for submitting a bid and includes:

- Name, telephone number, and address of the contact person or RFP director
- Basic submission requirements, including
  —number of proposal copies needed
  —deadline for submission
  —dates of bidders' conferences
  —how and when the winning bidder will be notified
  —security issues
  —restrictions
  —required format
- Notification that proposals written in response to the RFP may be incorporated into the subsequent contract between the health care organization and the vendor, and that any false or misleading statements in a proposal are grounds for disqualification
- Notice that consideration will be given only to those proposals that have clear, economical writing, use simple charts, and comply with the instructions for submission of the RFP
- Anything else the team deems necessary to facilitate the review process for its health care organization

Qualifications

The qualifications section should request information on a company's background, finances, philosophy, and relevant experience. To ensure the ability to compare bidders on an apples-to-apples basis, the particulars of these requests, such as limiting relevant experience to the previous five years, should be dictated.

Project Management and Staffing

This section is especially important for RFPs that are service-related or involve products that require training and sophisticated installation.

(Some of the details of this section of the RFP may not be applicable to small-scale outsourcing needs.) Project management should be divided into the following four sections:

- *Project management approach.* Request a description of the method to be used to manage the project, and suggest information on details such as the use of on-site offices and subcontractors. Request a project management organizational structure, including reporting levels and lists of duties.
- *Project control.* The vendor should describe methods used to control the project activities, such as weekly staff and/or subcontractor meetings, and provide an outline of the planned distribution of meeting minutes.
- *Project schedule.* Long-term, multitask outsourced projects should have a timetable. A chart of project progression from start to completion, including dates for major milestones and project completion, should be prepared for the vendor. If the project is highly complex and requires wide-ranging coordination, information on the vendor's scheduling capabilities and computerized scheduling program should be requested to assist in the preparation of this chart.
- *Status reporting.* Information on the vendor's methods for reporting progress and issuing status reports on financial and logistical matters should be requested.

Project staffing is just as important as project management. Ultimately, services to be outsourced are delivered by people. Condensed resumes of key project personnel listed in the project management organizational structure should be requested. To protect against a vendor switching personnel after winning the bid, bidders should be reminded that the proposed personnel may be interviewed in the later stages of the proposal review process.

Functional Requirements

This section of the RFP should provide a logical breakdown of the requirements of the proposed outsourced project and list them in order of importance. Nonnegotiable issues should be in boldface and described as hard stops for vendors. For instance, the RFP might state that the materials management software must be able to export information to a spreadsheet for analysis. If vendors cannot meet this requirement, they need not respond.

If an outsourcing project is technical in nature, the functional requirements for the project may be complex and lengthy. In such a case, the functional requirements section of the RFP should include a vendor response survey, listing the needs of the project and providing "yes" and "no" boxes for bidders to check or multiple-choice answers. In effect, the survey allows the selection committee to review key information among the competing bidders easily. A well-conceived vendor response survey for computer or telecommunications functions may have more than 200 questions. See figures 7-1 and 7-2 for examples of RFP questions and a sample scoring system for outsourcing a clinical project.

Evaluation Criteria

An RFP should inform the bidders of the way the winning bid will be determined. However, it is a matter of discretion as to how much of the evaluation method is revealed. Generally, bidders are informed that the criteria are the completeness of the response to the RFP and the ability of the bidder to meet objectives and requirements. However, the operations team may want to request specifics in the bids received, such as price or on-site management, in this section.

Glossary of Terms

A glossary of terms is a good idea for RFPs that deal with technologies or services that are relatively new and do not have an industry-accepted vernacular. For example, PC-based inventory systems must be adequately defined by the health care organization so that vendors cannot misconstrue the concept. This would include potential network needs and whether the systems are real time or batch-processed download dumps to the mainframe. If a number of different vendors propose solutions with differing terminology, the process of evaluating the proposals becomes more complex. A glossary of terms lessens the possibility of confusion on the bidders' part.

FIGURE 7-1. Sample RFP Questions: Bone Densitometry Services

1. How will the equipment be acquired for this program?

   Capital purchase by health care facility
   Capital purchase by vendor
   Lease by health care facility
   Lease by vendor
   Risk-share program

2. If technology should change, will there be any additional charge for the program?

   Yes
   No

3. Will there be annual price increases in the contract?

   Yes
   No

   If yes, please indicate the percentage of increase: Will this be a fixed increase annually?

   Yes
   No

   If no, what will be the basis of the increase?

4. Who will provide the clinical staff for this program?

   Health care facility
   Vendor

5. What will the educational requirements be for the clinical staff provided by the vendor?

   High school diploma
   Advanced degree
   Undergraduate degree
   Clinical training
   Other

6. Who will provide the professional staff (i.e., physicians) for this program?

   Health care facility
   Vendor

FIGURE 7-1. (Continued)

7. What clinical discipline will these individuals be drawn from?

   Gynecology
   Orthopedics
   Internal medicine
   Radiology
   Other

8. What will the hours of operation be?

   Day shift (8 AM to 4 PM)
   Evening shift 1 to 2 nights a week
   Evening shift nightly
   Saturday mornings
   Saturday afternoons
   Other (please specify)

9. How many operational hours a week do you guarantee?

   0 to 20
   21 to 35
   36 to 50
   51 or more

10. Who will be responsible for the completion of reports?

    Health care facility
    Vendor

11. If the vendor, what is the guaranteed turnaround time?

12. If the vendor, how will these reports be generated?

    On-site via PC
    Off-site via PC
    Off-site by outside vendor

FIGURE 7-2. Sample RFP Scoring System: Bone Densitometry Services

Use of a scoring system is sometimes advisable. Weighting of particular questions is dependent on the goals of an organization. This RFP is for bone densitometry. The organization is looking for a team that will be totally responsible for a program, including clinical staff and report generation. Physicians are to be supplied by the hospital. Demand for the service is moderate to high, with most patients requesting evening and Saturday appointments.

To calculate scores, add points for each answer. Vendors with the highest scores should be interviewed before the "winner" is selected. (This scoring system should not be shared with vendors.)

1. How will the equipment be acquired for this program?
   Capital purchase by health care facility (+3)
   Capital purchase by vendor (+5)
   Lease by heath care facility (+1)
   Lease by vendor (+4)
   Risk-share program (+6)

2. If technology should change, any additional charge for the program?
   Yes (–2)
   No (+2)

   If yes, please estimate the increase:
   0 to 2.5% (+4)
   2.5 to 4% (+3)
   4 to 8% (0)
   >8% (–4)
   Flat $ fee (+1)

3. Will there be annual price increases in the contract?
   Yes (–3)
   No (+3)
   Amount of increase
      0 to 2.5% (+4)
      2.5 to 4% (+3)
      4 to 8% (0)
      >8% (–4)
   Fixed increase (–2)
      Tied to CPI (–4)
      Tied to health care CPI (+4)

FIGURE 7-2. (Continued)

4. What will the hours of operation be?
   Day shift (8 AM to 4 PM) (+2)
   Evening shift 1 to 2 nights a week (+4)
   Evening shift nightly (+5)
   Saturday mornings (+4)
   Saturday afternoons (+4)
   Other (+1)

5. How many hours a week are guaranteed?
   0 to 20 (+1)
   21 to 35 (+3)
   36 to 50 (+5)
   51 or more (−2)

6. Who will be responsible for the completion of reports?
   Health care facility (+3)
   Vendor (+1)

7. If the vendor, what is the guaranteed turnaround time?
   0 to 2 hours (+1)
   2 to 8 hours (+1)
   8 to 24 hours (+5)
   Over 24 hours (+1)

8. If the vendor, how will these reports be generated?
   On-site via PC (+1)
   Off-site via PC (+5)
   Off-site by outside vendor (+3)

9. Who will provide the clinical staff for this program?*
   Health care facility (+4)
   Vendor (0)

10. Educational requirements for the clinical staff provided by the vendor?*
    High school diploma (+1)
    Undergraduate degree (+3)
    Advanced degree (+1)
    Clinical training (+5)
    Other (0)

(Continued on next page)

FIGURE 7-2.   (Continued)

11. Who will provide the professional staff (i.e., physicians) for this program?*
    Health care facility (+4)
    Vendor (0)

12. What clinical discipline will these individuals be drawn from if provided by the vendor?*
    Gynecology (+2)
    Orthopedics (+3)
    Internal medicine (+1)
    Radiology (+1)
    Other (0)

Total_____

*Scores may depend on goals of institution

Description of Vendor

The health care organization should request information from the vendor that would provide a clear picture of its operation, including:

- Financial stability
- Quality of staff
- Quality control efforts
- Reputation within the industry
- Experience
- Rate of growth
- Philosophy and mission (to determine cultural fit)

References

A complement to the qualifications section, this portion of the RFP should request the contact names and phone numbers of ten references. References should be requested for individual project staff members as well as the firm in general. For large and complex projects, insurance and bank references and audited financial statements should be solicited as well.

Fees and Costs

To ensure an easy comparison among bidders, the full spectrum of services and/or products needed should be outlined in this section, and line-item costs and fees requested. If the RFP is a solutions proposal and does not list costs and fees for the bidders, they should be asked to be as detailed as possible in their breakdown of costs and to include a statement that any costs not itemized by them will be their responsibility. Also, bidders should be asked to detail the payment terms and any performance clauses that they would expect.

Appendices

This closing section of the RFP allows the operations team to include any information that would facilitate a bidder's understanding of the proposed outsourcing project. For example, an RFP for market research services might include a previous market research project undertaken by the health care organization and a cover note explaining its merits and faults. Another example: an RFP for information services might include a graphic of the existing computer network to ensure adherence to the existing infrastructure.

ISSUING REQUESTS FOR PROPOSAL

The operations team should issue an RFP only to firms highly qualified to submit the bid and do the work. (Developing a list of firms was covered in chapter 6.) To ensure that only certain types of vendors respond to an RFP, a cover letter should be attached describing the qualities sought in the vendor. The cover letter can act as a preview to the qualifications and functional requirements sections of the RFP and will allow certain vendors to rule themselves out.

Both bidders' conferences and site visits (discussed in chapter 6) are advised for large, complex, and expensive RFPs, such as substantial construction projects or important services such as food and nutrition. A bidders' conference is a meeting called by the health care organization at which all of the vendors who are bidding on a project can ask questions about the RFP and clarify issues. This arrangement allows the health care organization to keep the playing field level and provides each vendor with an opportunity to discuss any concerns or reservations about the proposal.

EVALUATING PROPOSALS

The real work starts when the RFPs are returned. The operations team is now charged with ensuring that vendors followed instructions. The next step is to analyze each of the proposals for required components.

Initial Evaluation

The fulfillment of the basic requirements of the RFP provides the basis for the initial evaluation of proposals. The basics include meeting the deadline for submission, providing the correct number of copies, adhering to the suggested format, and, of course, pricing within budgetary parameters. Vendors who do not meet basic requirements or submit sloppy proposals are probably poor candidates and should be disqualified unless extenuating circumstances dictate otherwise.

Short List and In-Depth Review

A short list of potential vendors should be established as quickly as possible so that the operations team can begin a more rigorous, in-depth review. In addition to firms that do not meet the basic requirements, other firms will disqualify themselves with poor presentations. A cursory review of the proposals often results in a manageable short list.

The next level of evaluation requires that proposals be read carefully and, if a point scoring system is in place, scored at this point. The selection team members may divide the proposals among themselves, or each member may read all the proposals. In any case, reviewers should be alert to the fulfillment of the major issues of the RFP. Other issues to check for are a demonstration of the firm's ability to perform as stated in the RFP; the believability of the proposal and its schedule;

the reasonableness of its costs and fees; and the adequacy of the firm's references, related experience, personnel, and financial stability. Exceptions to items in the RFP should be allowed if a vendor presents an alternative proposal and provides a suitable explanation for its novel approach.

Following this more intensive review, a group of finalists should emerge as firms distinguish themselves with excellent overall proposals. The operations team may check the point scoring system again at this stage in the review process, when the characteristics that distinguish the competing bidders are less obvious and the proposals need to be reevaluated.

SELECTING A WINNING BID

If the short list is long and competitive, a second round of elimination may be necessary. In the case of expensive, complex outsourcing projects, an interview of the vendor's personnel or a demonstration of the vendor's product is recommended. Both of these activities should be figured into the evaluation point scoring system and each merit a considerable percentage of the score, perhaps 25 percent. (The scoring can be compared to an educational grading system; for example, 50 percent of a grade may derive from the term paper, 25 percent from the final, and 25 percent from class participation.)

When the review process is complete, the operations team issues a recommendation to the decision maker, who is most likely the CEO or COO. The team's recommendation is based on both objective and subjective measures. Even when an outsourcing project consists mainly of the procurement of a capital expense, such as a magnetic resonance imaging machine, there are always the human elements of service and training to be considered. Therefore, the team members should keep in mind that as helpful as scoring systems are in making a solid decision about technology, intuition is usually the best guide in making decisions about people.

Ultimately, a successful RFP is a document that results in an excellent relationship with a vendor or partner. As in any good relationship, communication between the parties must be clear and timely. Because an RFP often represents the first significant communication between health care organization and vendor, the document ought to be carefully and strategically crafted. Likewise, the effort expended by the vendor in responding ought to be considered.

The following list of questions should help your operations team develop an effective RFP:

- Should an outside consultant be used?
- Which team member is ultimately responsible for the RFP?
- What are the goals of the RFP?
- What are the elements of the RFP?
- Is it appropriate to use a standard RFP?
- Who should receive an RFP and the invitation to bid the project?
- Are vendor meetings and site visits appropriate within the RFP process?
- What are the criteria for initially evaluating a bid?
- How is a short list of proposals for review selected?
- What is the process for selecting bidders?
- What is the process for determining winners?
- Who will make the final decision on winners?

CONCLUSION

An RFP is a legal, technical, and business document that requires a principal author and organizer, but cannot be accomplished without a team effort. Health care organizations that execute an RFP in the context of a focused approach to outsourcing have a number of advantages over those that simply identify a business need or problem and proceed to write an RFP. The outsourcing process that precedes the writing of an RFP provides the authors of the document with an excellent foundation upon which to build a comprehensive and detailed explanation of a health care organization's needs.

Reference

1. K. D. Schwartz. NIST's Model RFP Helps Unravel Mystery of Contracts, *Government Computer News* 12, no. 13 (June 1993): 64.

8

Drafting an Outsourcing Contract

T he outsourcing agreement legally binds the vendor to provide the services required by the department being outsourced. The request for proposal should provide a basic outline of the scope of services required and should be used as a guideline in preparing the contract for the vendor. Using the RFP as the basis of the contract should:

- Increase the likelihood that key operations are included
- Reduce the chance of unforeseen consequences
- Incorporate complete disclosure of expectations
- Provide the basis for performance monitoring and conflict resolution

Some organizations have found themselves in the lurch because key elements were omitted from the contract. In such cases, a vendor may be either unwilling to accept additional responsibilities or only willing to accept them for an additional fee. Therefore, the contract must be structured precisely so that all aspects of the service being outsourced are presented to the vendor.

Although the vendor selection process is generally a team effort, the writing of the contract itself should be handled by only one key individual, typically a member of the purchasing staff. After the contract is written, operations team members should review it for accidental omissions. The legal staff should perform the final review to ensure that the organization's interests are fully protected. The contract then should be effective as a management tool to evaluate vendor performance and as a basis for the relationship between the vendor and health care organization in the future.

This chapter reviews the elements that should be included in a well-written outsourcing contract for a nonclinical department. It also provides guidelines for addressing quality of care issues and performance criteria in an outsourcing contract for a clinical department.

TRENDS IN OUTSOURCING CONTRACTS

Today's outsourcing contracts must be very specific and detailed to ensure that the vendor's performance meets the needs of the institution. Two basic elements of a traditional contract have changed: price and duration.

Price

Over the past decade, profit margins of vendors have been squeezed a number of times. As hospital reimbursement decreased as a result of prospective payment and managed care, health care managers demanded that suppliers of goods and services cut their prices. Prices are unlikely to drop further; instead, new savings will come from the efficient and cost-effective use of systems and technologies. Thus, rather than price, today's vendors are more likely to focus their sales pitch on how their service differs from and improves on the service offered by their competition. The advantage to the health care organization of this approach is that the service offered by a potential vendor can be structured to fit the needs of the institution.

Duration

Vendors prefer to invest in longer-term contracts. Therefore, it is appropriate to specify a contract duration of at least three years. But what happens if the relationship does not work out for some reason?

Previously, outsourcing contracts contained an outclause that allowed the organization to discontinue using a vendor. In today's contracts, outclauses have been replaced by "just cause" clauses, which detail specific reasons when and why an agreement can be terminated.

Their focus is much narrower than that of outclauses in the past because of the larger scope of the investment required of the vendor. To make the outlay worthwhile, the reasons that the contract can be terminated should be narrowly defined. For example, if a long-term care facility has outsourced its rehabilitation activities, the vendor will have a significant investment in personnel and equipment. An abrupt termination of the contract could prove detrimental to its viability. Specific reasons that this contract might be terminated would include use of nonlicensed therapists or a lack of appropriate treatment regimens for specific patients.

STANDARD SECTIONS OF AN OUTSOURCING CONTRACT

Every contract contains certain essential elements. These include:

- Basic structure
- Fees
- Price increases
- Performance criteria
- Incentives and penalties
- Transition plans
- Contingency plans
- Indemnification
- Ownership of methodologies
- Definition of the partnership
- Management of human resources

Figure 8-1 is a sample outsourcing contract.

Basic Structure

The first section of the agreement should specify who provides what service to whom. Although this may sound simplistic, it is vital to ensure that there is no misunderstanding regarding the expectations of the health care organization or the vendor in the future.

FIGURE 8-1. Sample Outsourcing Contract*

Introduction

This is an agreement between Community Hospital (Hospital), a non-profit health care facility and Bone Services (Company), a private corporation, for the provision of bone densitometry services. The Company will assume responsibility for the scheduling, performance, interpretation, results reporting and invoicing of all outpatient studies performed at the Hospital. This agreement will be in effect from January 1, 1999, through December 31, 2002. The Company may not perform any other diagnostic or therapeutic procedure on the Hospital campus without prior approval of the Hospital.

The Hospital and the Company are two separate organizations. Each is responsible to maintain appropriate levels of malpractice insurance for the completion of its responsibilities. Each party agrees to "hold harmless" the other entity provided that any actions are prudent.

Payments

Space in the Hospital will be rented by the Company at a cost of $5/square foot/month. The current configuration of allocated space totals 200 square feet, resulting in a monthly payment by the Company to the Hospital of $1,000. Increases in the rent payment will be annually on January 1st, at a rate equal to the Consumer Price Index (CPI) (non-health care).

All equipment, staffing and supplies required to perform this service are the sole responsibility of the Company. Supplies may be purchased from the hospital at a rate of cost plus 50%. Any applicable taxes will be the responsibility of the Company.

Performance Criteria

Because this agreement covers services delivered to patients of the Hospital, there is a need to establish performance criteria. The following standards will be in effect throughout the life of the contract:

1. The hours of operation for bone densitometry service will be 8 AM to 5 PM Monday through Friday and 8 AM through 12 noon on Saturdays. No hours will be available on Sundays.

2. There will be two evenings a month in which appointments may be scheduled. Hours shall be 5 PM through 9 PM. Requests for these appointment slots will be monitored. At least once every six months, appointment availability will be reviewed for a determination of whether evening hours should be expanded. This decision

FIGURE 8-1. (Continued)

will be made jointly between authorized representatives of the Hospital and the Company.

3. Average wait time for an appointment slot should not exceed 5 days.

4. Turnaround time on dictated reports will not exceed 24 hours.

5. Exams will be interpreted by a qualified medical professional who will be approved by the medical staff board.

Penalties

In the event that the performance of bone densitometry studies cannot be provided due to staffing problems, equipment downtime, or lack of professional staff to interpret studies, the Company shall pay the Hospital $100/day for every day that the situation continues.

Resolution of Problems

In the event that during the life of this agreement, issues or disputes arise that cannot be amicably resolved, the Hospital and the Company will submit the issue to the Hospital President for resolution. Both parties agree to submit to this procedure and to abide by the decision of the President.

Transition Period

The Hospital does not currently provide this service for patients. Therefore, a period of no longer than 90 days will be provided to the vendor for the purpose of hiring staff and acquiring all needed equipment. During this time period, the identified space within the Hospital will be renovated as discussed in the document titled "Space Renovation," dated June 15, 1998.

Patients will be able to schedule appointments starting January 1, 1999; however, only 50% of the total appointment slots will be available. Full capacity will be available as of March 1, 1999.

Unresolved Problems

In the event that an impasse between the Hospital and the Company develops and the agreement is to be terminated, the following phase-out process will be implemented:

1. Staff employed by the Company at the Hospital site may be interviewed by the Hospital for potential employment after the contract is terminated.

(Continued on next page)

FIGURE 8-1.   (Continued)

2. Company equipment at the site will be evaluated for purchase by the Hospital, providing that the Company provides documentation of the age and book value of said equipment.

3. A 90-day period during which the Hospital will develop and implement a plan to either assume control of bone densitometry services or to acquire another vendor will be established.

4. All prepaid rental payments, less any penalties, will be returned to the Company.

5. Any work procedures, forms, or methodologies used in the performance of the patient studies will become the property of the Hospital.

The termination of this contract would be detrimental to both the Hospital and the Company. Therefore, the reasons that the contract can be terminated have been narrowed to include the following:

• Arrears in rental payment that are greater than 6 months with no plan to resolve
• Ongoing lack of appointment times resulting in waits of 10 days or more
• Delays in report distribution equal to or exceeding 96 hours in three consecutive months

Mergers and Acquisitions

In the event that the Hospital acquires other health care facilities or is acquired by another organization, this agreement will remain in effect for a period of 6 months. During this time, the Hospital and the Company will explore their relationship and whether it can be expanded, remain intact, or be terminated.

*This sample contract demonstrates how elements identified in the steps of the outsourcing process are incorporated. It is not meant to replace or substitute for contracts written by a purchasing department of a health care organization or by its general counsel.

Also included in this section is information regarding the vendor: is it a private or a public company, is it a wholly-owned subsidiary of another firm, what is the relationship between the subsidiary and the parent organization? This information may prove to be valuable to the hospital if a problem should arise or if the vendor is unable to provide the contracted services or respond satisfactorily to a hospital's inquiries.

Fees

For most managers, fees are considered the most important element of the contract. Fee structures today may look different from those of the past. Currently, there are four basic fee structures:

- *Fixed fee structure* is a flat fee for a specified time frame and is generally set at a level to ensure cost savings. A fixed fee structure may be useful in situations where volume and activity are fairly stable. In the past, 61 percent of contracts were written using this structure.[1]
- *Variable fee structure* changes based on the actual time spent on a project. Variable fees would be useful in those situations where the level of activity fluctuates. For example, if a small facility outsources its computer maintenance function, a flat fee structure would be inappropriate because there will be times when no work is required from the vendor. In this case, pricing based on actual hours that the computer staff works on a hospital's systems would be the most appropriate.
- *Volume fee structure* is another variable structure based on a volume of activity—often patient volume. This structure might be used when a department like physical therapy is outsourced. The hospital will pay a per-patient fee for every patient who is treated in the vendor's facility. With proper record keeping and analysis, appropriate per-patient fees can be determined and the hospital can match revenues and expenses.
- *Mixed fee structure* is a combination of two or more of the fee structures mentioned above. For instance, in outsourcing a department or function that, in general, has a steady stream of business but experiences seasonal increases, a flat fee per month could be established with a provision for an additional volume fee to be incorporated into the contract when volume reaches or exceeds a certain stated amount.

Price Increases

Once a fee structure has been chosen, annual or inflationary influences must be considered and addressed in detail in the contract. In some instances, the vendor will push for a flat, percentage increase in all subsequent years, often at a rate higher than inflation. A more cost-effective method of setting price increases is to stipulate that increases will equal the annual increase as measured by the overall consumer price index (CPI). This will ensure that the contract price is adjusted fairly. It should be noted that using the health care CPI, an index that directly ties to prices within the health care industry, is not recommended, since this index may be adjusted for a variety of reasons (for example, fiscal policy or reimbursement trends), which may not be applicable to the outsourcing contract.

Performance Criteria

Baseline for performance must be included in the contract so that the vendor is required to meet expectations. In some cases, vendors may explain that the text of their sales brochures covers such issues. Whether such brochures include information about performance levels is irrelevant. If the expectations are not included in the contract, there will be no legal basis on which to hold the vendor responsible.

These standards should not be difficult to develop, as they will have been identified in the early stages of the outsourcing process. Performance indicators used to evaluate the current level of performance and included in the RFP will be included in the contract. Performance standards should define current performance of department/function and outline how it should be improved over time. If such criteria are not included, there is no basis on which to judge the vendor's performance. Performance criteria might include average wait for appointments in an imaging center, turnaround time for telephone requests for supplies (hospital distribution), or number of errors on patient bills in a physician's office.

Incentives and Penalties

Once the performance criteria have been included in the contract, inclusion of related penalties and incentives is easy. These can be directly tied to the revenue enhancement or cost reduction that the vendor achieves; vendors may be rewarded for timeliness or penalized for slow implementation of elements, or incentives and penalties may be tied to quality indicators or performance criteria. Examples include:

- The vendor will receive 50 percent of all cost reductions exceeding $500,000.
- The vendor will receive $25,000 if the management information system is installed and working within two months rather than four.
- The vendor will be penalized $100 every time an equipment request is not filled within one hour.

These clauses are designed to create incentives for the vendor to commit to the organization or penalize the vendor if responsibilities of the contract are not met.

Following are some specific issues to consider when designating reward/penalty clauses in an outsourcing contract to avoid confusion and disagreement in the future.

Measurement Criteria.   One specific reward/penalty issue to address in the contract is whether the performance criterion on which the reward or penalty is based can be accurately measured. This can be problematic. For instance, if the performance standard is that patients will be transported so as to arrive at appointments for diagnostic studies at least 15 minutes before the appointed time, there must be a mechanism to measure this. If the facility has a bar code system to sign patients in and out of areas, there may not be a problem. But if, like many health care organizations, there is a reliance on manual entries by transport staff, there may be a debate about accuracy of entries. Any performance criterion should be detailed in the contract along with the means for measuring it.

Performance Evaluation.   Another issue to resolve is when performance is to be judged and by whom. While it sounds trivial, some outsourcing firms price contracts believing that incentives can be easily obtained. Therefore, they will push for frequent measurement and awarding of bonuses. Conversely, if the vendor has a short-term problem that may affect performance, it may prefer less frequent performance measurement until the problem is fixed so as to avoid penalties. By designating a judge to provide evaluations and establishing a timetable, the health care organization will have more control over the awarding of bonuses and penalties.

Risk-Sharing Determination.   In the event there are savings generated through the outsourcing agreement, there should be an equitable means of assigning them to either the health care organization or the vendor or both. One means of doing this is to examine the amount of risk each party carries. If the responsibility is shared equally, risk is said to be shared, and savings (or revenue enhancement) should be shared equally. If the vendor assumes the bulk of effort in generating savings (or enhancing revenue), risk is said to be shifted and any benefits should flow to the vendor. The method chosen will depend on the service or activity involved and the ability to measure outcomes of any program.

Transition Plans

Plans for transition periods are often omitted from contracts. It is unclear whether the reason for this is because no one feels the need to spell out the plan or because the parties are so eager to move forward that they forgot to map out how. Regardless, a plan must be developed for the periods during which the contract is implemented and terminated.

Implementation Plan.   As the contract is signed, the parties must have a plan for transfer of responsibility and/or assets. This plan should be included in the contract to ensure that there is agreement, understanding, and commitment. Implementation will normally take a few weeks to a few months. This interval allows the vendor to review operations one last time, hire staff required by the contract, acquire any needed capital items, and orient the staff from both organizations to the new system. In more complicated contracts, the transition period allows gradual transfer of responsibility, particularly where the vendor will assume control over many functions.

For instance, if all forms of transportation are outsourced to one vendor, it may be helpful to implement the contract gradually by type of transportation. The vendor may start by assuming responsibility for in-house movement of supplies; then add mail, specimens, equipment, pharmaceuticals, and patients; and, finally, add off-campus movement of items. This gradual transfer of control can prove invaluable in

STANDARD SECTIONS OF AN OUTSOURCING CONTRACT

cementing a long-term and trusting relationship. In the case of assets, the agreement should specify when ownership changes hands and how payment will occur. (After the transfer of ownership occurs, the health care institution should evaluate whether there can or should be changes to maintenance agreements or insurance policies.)

Termination Plan.   There will be times that outsourcing relationships are dissolved, whether because of nonperformance or changes in strategic thinking. In such cases, there must be a formal plan outlining how the transition will be handled. Transfer of responsibility may be back to the health care facility or to another outsourcing vendor. The termination plan should include agreements on ownership of methodologies that may have been implemented by the vendor, ownership of equipment and other capital items, and steps that must be taken to ensure a smooth transition.

Perhaps most important, there should be a clear statement as to what fees may be owed to the vendor. This is especially important in the event that the contract is terminated prematurely. A transition plan is essential to ensure that the function is continued even if the vendor loses the contract. Some vendors have been known to pull their staff and equipment when told of a contract loss. Including a termination plan in the original contract may not prevent the firm from doing this, but it should spell out what will happen if the plan is not followed.

Contingency Plans

In addition to a section on transition plans, the contract should include one on contingency plans that cover emergencies or other unusual situations. Such conditions include natural disasters (for instance, blizzards, floods, and earthquakes), facility breakdowns (fire, for example), labor strife (such as a work stoppage), and merger or acquisition of the organization.

Natural Disasters.   A contingency plan with regard to natural disasters should spell out the roles of both the health care organization and the vendor. It should include designation of the outsource staff as either essential or nonessential personnel in such a circumstance. Inclusion of this information in the contract will help prevent misunderstandings during crucial events.

Labor Strife.   In the event of a work stoppage, the outsourcing contract should specify the expectations of each party. For example, should one labor group within the hospital strike, will the vendor continue to provide service (i.e., will the outsource staff cross picket lines)? A second concern is whether the vendor can be expected to "fill in" as necessary to ensure delivery of patient care. Outlining such issues in the agreement can alleviate problems that might otherwise cripple the organization.

Merger or Acquisition.   In today's health care environment, the chances of merger or acquisition are fairly high. If a health care organization is acquired by another entity, a clause in the contract must spell out the responsibilities of both partners as well as a statement of financial responsibilities. A number of organizations have found themselves unable to dissolve outsourcing agreements without large financial penalties. Conversely, some organizations have discovered that the agreements cannot be extended to the facilities that are acquired. Such situations should be anticipated and a resolution plan in place that would prevent financial losses.

Indemnification

The outsourcing agreement should contain a clause that neither party will or can hold the other responsible for certain actions. Called a "hold harmless" clause, this eliminates the ability of either group to point fingers at the other in the event of legal action. This section should explain the relationship between the vendor and its parent company (if one exists). In addition, it should outline the circumstances under which the parent will offer financial or other support to the subsidiary. These issues must be spelled out in the contract. Doing so will protect the interests of both the health care organization and the vendor.

Ownership of Methodologies

Ownership of any methodologies that have been implemented throughout the contract must be specified. This may include computer programs, work methods, structure, and so on. In addition, there may be techniques or ways and means identified while the contract is in effect, especially in academic settings, that may be useful for research and educational purposes. Specifying who owns such methodologies will prove useful if the contract is terminated.

Definition of the Partnership

The outsourcing contract should include a section that focuses on the relationship between the two parties. Defining this relationship in the legal agreement gives it weight and may help to resolve disputes. A number of issues should be addressed, including management, confidentiality, volume, technology, and disputes.

Management. How much autonomy the vendor's staff can have in making daily operating decisions should be spelled out, along with situations that would require consultation with the health care organization. For example, can the vendor change the hours of operation of a department?

Confidentiality. It is important that guidelines are developed for use of information and its dissemination and safeguarding. In addition, requirements of managed care increase the importance of information management. The role of the outsource vendor in maintaining records should be included in the outsourcing contract. If the vendor has access to patient names, the importance of confidentiality must be delineated in the contract.

Volume. Volume associated with any contract probably will vary. While small changes may have no effect on the outsourcing agreement, there should be a plan to deal with large increases or decreases in volume. If a service is added that affects the vendor, how will the contract be updated?

Technology. It is important to specify who decides when technology will be upgraded. In addition, when technology upgrades are necessary, provisions should be included in the contract for additional charges. If an updated software package becomes available, will the vendor assume the cost?

Dispute Resolution. Perhaps the most important item in this section is how disputes will be resolved. If this is not specified, there may be no way to reconcile differences. The choice of resolution strategy depends on a number of factors, such as the culture of the organization, the type of outsourced function, and the importance of the task to the institution. Outlining which strategy is selected and how it is to be employed must be included in the agreement so that any disputes that arise can be dealt with quickly and effectively. There are several methods to choose from, including the following:

- *Compromise with an inside facilitator:* The compromise method uses a third party who is an internal individual not involved in the outsourcing agreement. The third party listens to the position of each side and then renders a decision based on the perceived need or problem.
- *Mediation:* Mediation uses an outside third party to resolve a dispute, but parties are not bound to accept the decision of the third party. It is a totally voluntary process that may or may not succeed. The determining factors are the two parties involved—if they are not willing to consider a resolution offered by the outside mediator, there is no mandate to do so.
- *Arbitration:* Arbitration is a negotiated process whereby two parties agree to submit contract disputes to a third party and to accept the arbitrator's decision as final and binding.[2] This process is less formal than a court proceeding, but many managers dislike it because they feel as though they lose control of the process.
- *A legal proceeding:* The dispute is submitted to a judge who determines if there was a breach of contract. This is the most expensive and lengthy process.

Management of Human Resources

The final section to consider for inclusion in the contract deals with current and future human resources. This is important because once an agreement is implemented and employees are transferred, a health care organization will have no control over how staff is treated by the vendor. At a minimum, the contract should address staffing levels, disposition of current staff, hiring of staff, and disposition of staff if the contract is dissolved.

Staffing Levels.   The role of the health care organization in determining staffing levels should be outlined. It would be unreasonable to assume that staffing levels used in the past would continue unchanged in the future. Most outsourcing vendors develop standard training methods and work principles so that staffing levels can be lowered. However, the health care organization must safeguard the quality of the service or function delivered. If staffing falls below certain levels, it can affect performance and the public's perception of service. Therefore, a health care organization should insist on some role in determining the level of staffing.

Disposition of Current Staff.   The contract should include provisions for the placement of current staff. If there is a collective bargaining agreement currently in place, it may spell out the options. Even in this case, however, the outsourcing contract also should specify what happens to employees. Options to be considered are early retirement, assimilation into the vendor ranks, assimilation into other vacant positions within the health care organization, or a workforce reduction. Although it would appear that these issues would be settled before the agreement takes effect, it is possible that individuals on the hospital payroll would be transferred to the vendor and eliminated later. Methods of dealing with this issue should be included in the contract.

Hiring Staff.   Although this is rarely problematic, the ability of one organization to hire staff from the other should be outlined. Many times this applies to the health care organization, eliminating their ability to hire the outsource staff to perform an activity internally. However, in some instances the vendor may seek certain individuals employed by the hospital in order to expand their offerings or meet the needs of another client. Therefore, the rights of each party should be defined in the outsourcing document.

Disposition of Staff If Contract Is Dissolved.   There should be provisions in the agreement delineating staff disposition in the event that the contract/relationship is dissolved. This should indicate whether individuals previously employed by the health care organization could be asked to return in such cases.

OUTSOURCING CONTRACT FOR CLINICAL SERVICES

When the focus of an outsourcing agreement is a clinical service, the contract requirements are similar to those of a nonclinical service, but must also include the qualifications of the staff involved and the quality of the service provided. Issues to be addressed include quality of care, credentialing, regulatory agency compliance, managed care requirements, and more.

Quality of Care

The level of patient care that is expected of the vendor's staff must be specified. Requirements will flow directly from the RFP, which asked for particular standards. For example, turnaround time for equipment deliveries requested in the RFP becomes the standard for the contract. The contract should also detail when and how often performance is measured against the standards.

In addition to measuring vendor performance, patient and/or physician satisfaction should also be measured. For example, feedback from satisfaction surveys may be the basis for measuring a vendor's performance in dietary services.

Credentialing

Whenever clinicians are involved, it is necessary to ensure that their preparation, training, licensure, and insurance information are accurate and up-to-date. Who performs the credentialing—the health care organization or the vendor—perhaps is less important than ensuring that the credentialing is done properly. However, if the credentialing is performed by the vendor, the outsourcing agreement must stipulate how the health care organization will be notified of any problems. Records pertaining to credentials should be readily available, making on-site storage attractive.

Regulatory Agency Compliance

Some areas of the health care organization must maintain records in order to comply with regulations of federal, state, and accrediting agencies. The outsourcing agreement should specify which party will maintain records and where and whether the outsource staff will be available to answer inquiries during inspections. Examples of records that should be maintained are safety inspections, testing logs, and minutes of meetings.

Managed Care Requirements

Managed care organizations (MCOs) have placed increased demands on health care organizations for information tracking and management. Which party is responsible for performing these activities, as well as who will interface with the MCO, should be spelled out in the outsourcing contract.

Miscellaneous Issues

Clinical outsourcing contracts should consider a number of other issues, including:

- *Benchmarking:* For example, wait time in ED as calculated by the state department of health
- *Financial reporting:* For example, cost per surgical procedure for outsourced anesthesia department
- *Participation on internal committees:* For example, the vendor of radiation therapy services must provide representation on the radiation safety committee
- *Participation on outside professional organizations:* For example, the staff of an outsourced skilled nursing unit must have representation on a long-term care professional association

CONCLUSION

Although it would certainly be easier to accept the contract written by the vendor, there is little reason to expect that such a document would protect the needs of the health care organization. Including all sections discussed in this chapter will help to ensure that the rights of each party are protected. The outsourcing contract, once written and signed, becomes a management tool. Rather than file it away, the manager should review requirements and set up mechanisms to ensure that conditions are met. In some instances, this process will be easy and require minimal effort on the part of the hospital staff. In other cases, there will be a need for detailed analysis and careful tracking of performance. This process is more fully explained in chapter 9, which describes the role of contract facilitator.

References

1. S. McEachern. Risk Shared Outsourcing Will Soar as Build-or-Buy Solution. *Healthcare Strategic Management* 14, no. 1 (January 1996).

2. M. R. Carrell and C. Heavrin. *Collective Bargaining* (Columbus, OH: Bell and Howell Co., 1985), pp. 326–28.

Additional Outsourcing Roles and Options

9

The Contract Facilitator

T
o ensure that both the hospital and the vendor achieve their goals, someone must monitor level of performance, ensure that milestones are reached, and facilitate open communication that allows for the resolution of problems. This is the role of the contract facilitator.

This chapter reviews various approaches that may be used in choosing a contract facilitator and explores the job responsibilities from both an internal and external perspective. In addition to explaining the function of a facilitator, this chapter clarifies how management can become involved at the appropriate level in response to specific outsourcing situations.

DEFINITION OF THE CONTRACT FACILITATOR POSITION

The contract facilitator is the person or persons held responsible for the implementation and ongoing maintenance of outsourcing contracts. This responsibility may be delegated to one individual internally, a group of internal managers or administrators, or an outside contractor. The choice depends on the complexity of the contract and the estimated time needed to ensure that the contract is fully operational. In the case of a limited activity for which one outside firm is to be chosen, the need for outside expertise and assistance is minimal. However, as the number, size, and complexity of activities outsourced in a contract grow, the health care organization may find it advantageous to consider an outside company to manage the contracts.

After the plan to outsource has been put into place, there will be a need for information over the life of the contract. To control the type and flow of information, the contract facilitator should consider the following questions:

- What information will be needed to implement the contract?
- What information will be needed on an ongoing basis?
- Who will need the information?
- How will that individual receive the information?
- Do other internal staff members need this information?
- How will they get it?
- How will the vendor get needed information?
- How will we know if there have been changes in technology or practice related to this service?
- How will we relate these changes to the vendor?
- When will information be exchanged?

PROCESS OF SELECTING A CONTRACT FACILITATOR

One of the last chores of the operations team before disbanding is to decide whether the proposed outsourcing contract will be managed internally or externally. If it is to be managed internally, the team may select a member to act as the contract facilitator. If the decision is made to look outside the organization, the team can recommend a small subgroup to evaluate prospective candidates for this position. This process requires an administrator with an understanding of the department activity being outsourced, one or two managers to interview the outsiders, and a finance person to review proposals. In some cases, the outsourcing process may have already identified a contract facilitator during previous projects, which will make the selection process easier.

Traits of a Contract Facilitator

An effective contract facilitator should be:

- Objective
- Open to new ideas
- Able to speak articulately

- Attentive to details
- Capable of sustaining long-term vision

Sources of Contract Facilitators

Basically, contract facilitators may be chosen from three sources: the purchasing department, an operations team member involved in the management of the outsourced department, or an outside consulting firm. Each offers advantages and disadvantages.

Purchasing Department.   Some health care organizations give the responsibility to oversee all contracts to the purchasing department, seeing no reason to change their approach for an outsourcing contract. The difficulty with such an approach is the volume of work that already falls on the shoulders of this busy department. Besides preparing most of the bids that are issued by an institution, the purchasing department must review all purchasing proposals, remain current with various types of corporate jargon and offerings, obtain bids on capital equipment, and update price changes to user departments. This does not permit the staff to invest the time needed to oversee complicated outsourcing contracts.

Some larger hospital organizations have expanded the role of the purchasing manager, whom they call the chief resource officer (CRO), to include contract negotiation and management of finances, human resources, capital resources, plant and equipment, and other assets of a facility. The CRO is charged with ensuring that all of these resources are used efficiently and effectively for the long term, with less emphasis on short-term savings than on strategic benefits.

Once outsourcing contracts are put into place for non-core services, the CRO's responsibility is to oversee the contract, ensuring that the expected levels of performance are met and other benefits achieved. In these cases, the CRO functions as the contract facilitator.

Management of an Outsourced Department.   Many health care organizations assign the contract facilitator responsibility to an experienced manager who is familiar with the outsourced area. For example, the director of respiratory therapy, a member of the team that developed a contract to outsource equipment repair, might be chosen to facilitate the contract for outsourcing respiratory therapy. However, as health care organizations continue to refocus internal energies on core competencies, even this approach may be problematic because it adds to the administrative load of the director.

Outside Consulting Firm.   A large outsourcing contract may require more involvement, especially at the outset, than an internal manager can offer. In such cases, some health care organizations may choose an outside firm to manage one or more of its outsourcing agreements. This frees up internal staff to manage their assigned departments and take advantage of the basic philosophy of outsourcing: if an activity is not a core competency that adds value to the organization's mission, have someone else do it. Experts are expected to oversee implementation, monitor performance, and provide updates to the health care organization.

CONTRACT FACILITATOR ROLE AND RESPONSIBILITIES

The basic responsibility of the contract facilitator is to ensure that outsourcing contracts are fulfilled. This may be an overwhelming challenge, since it involves both internal and external responsibilities. There may be involvement in the process before the contract is awarded, participation in developing the contracts, or merely follow-up monitoring after the contract is in place. Usually, the amount of involvement in each phase depends to a large degree on whether the facilitator is on board at the time.

Internal Responsibilities

Whether the contract facilitator is an employee of the health care organization or an outside consultant, this position requires involvement in internal responsibilities, including demand analysis, performance criteria identification, performance monitoring, and satisfaction assessment.

Demand Analysis.   As discussed in chapter 5, demand analysis allows for the projection of future needs. The facilitator need not know the ins-and-outs of every department, but should have the ability to ascertain what will be needed in terms of service levels through interviews and questionnaires. This work supplements, but does not replace, the committee approach to defining requirements as described in chapter 4. The facilitator should not be isolated from the staff or permitted to operate in a vacuum, since that can lead to potential conflicts of interest or ethical dilemmas.

Identification of Performance Criteria.   Identification of performance criteria by the facilitator will be used to judge the performance of the department under consideration. While a department or function may give the impression of efficiency, no definitive assessment of its performance can be made until the activity is compared with another organization's efforts. The facilitator, with the knowledge of internal workings and a network of resources from which to draw, should be called on to assist in establishing a benchmark checklist. Such a responsibility makes the outside firm, with a broader knowledge of health care organizations, attractive in the role as facilitator.

Performance Monitoring.   One of the facilitator's most important functions may be ensuring that the level of performance established and/or guaranteed in the outsourcing agreement is, in fact, achieved. This function may be the key to successful contracts in that if no one is responsible for ensuring that agreed-on standards are met, there may be a level of dissatisfaction that leads to nonrenewal of the contract. The facilitator has the task of ensuring that performance is monitored against that stated in the contract. If there are problems, the facilitator, through other roles described below, must step in to deal with them.

Satisfaction Assessment.   Even with continuous monitoring and communication, from time to time the contract may have a serious impact on the activities of departments and areas that are only remotely related to the outsourcing contract. The contract facilitator must pursue the concerns and address the issues raised by these departments, smooth out the rough areas of the contract, and ensure continuity of service within the health care organization.

External Responsibilities

In addition to internal tasks, the contract facilitator is responsible for a number of external tasks. These include coordinating the flow of information and doing industry research.

Coordinating the Flow of Information

Once an outsourcing contract is in place, information must flow between the health care organization and the vendor(s), including updates on program implementation, milestones, performance levels, problem areas, feedback from customers, and benchmarking. The contract facilitator must funnel such information between the vendor and the internal staff efficiently. The contract facilitator should ensure that the appropriate individuals receive needed information expeditiously in order to maintain optimum performance levels.

Doing Industry Research

To ensure that the levels of performance keep abreast of industry changes, the contract facilitator should be responsible for monitoring external trends. Changes within the health care industry can affect the expectations of the vendor and the organization. Research should include benchmarking activities, trends, regulatory changes, and new technology to ensure that the level of performance is in line with industry standards and to periodically update the contract.

CONCLUSION

The flow of information between health care organization and vendor is vital to the success of the outsourcing agreement. Internal and external changes may require alterations and adjustments in the contract, and the lack of an organized mechanism for the flow of information may result in gaps in understanding and miscommunication. Assigning the responsibility for information flow to an internal or external contract facilitator can prevent communication problems from occurring.

In some organizations, the need to ensure the accurate and timely flow of information and the appropriate allocation of resources has resulted in the creation of a chief resource officer position. While this position is appropriate for larger institutions, the need to ensure adequate and timely flow of information is vital to all institutions. Assigning the responsibility to a contract facilitator can safeguard the interests of both the health care organization and the outsource provider.

10
Communication

C ommunication is the cornerstone of success. After the contract is in place, many facilities turn their attention elsewhere, trusting the contractor to manage the agreement. However, maintaining strong, open, two-way communication through the life of the contract is essential to the success of the outsourcing arrangement.

This chapter describes how information can be communicated effectively to the health care organization's managers and employees and to the community at large. Because each of these groups has different needs that can shape the amount, type, and source of information they require from the vendor, establishing a mechanism to meet these needs early in the outsourcing process will ensure that the appropriate information is disseminated expeditiously, preventing misunderstandings that may hinder efficiency.

THE COMMUNICATOR ROLE

In chapter 9, information flow was identified as a key responsibility of the contract facilitator, who is expected to maintain lines of communication with the vendor. The purpose of such communication is to monitor the vendor's level of performance, ensure that the level of performance is in accordance with contract requirements, and to identify and resolve problems and issues before they affect the activities of the entire organization.

However, the contract facilitator, immersed in such daily activities, should not be expected to maintain the flow of communication to internal departments or the public. This responsibility should fall to an administrator or to the public relations department. By organizing the release of information, the communicator can protect the organization's image in the eyes of the staff and the public. For instance, in a scenario where a community hospital plans to outsource its coffee shop, an administrator should be given responsibility for communicating the expected changes internally, perhaps through the employee newsletter, and the public relations department might assume responsibility for announcing the change to the public through newspaper articles or interviews with local news organizations.

After staff members become aware of the outsourcing of a service, department, or function, their concern for their own futures becomes an issue. Questions are sure to arise not only from management and staff who are involved in the outsourced service directly, but also from those only peripherally involved or not involved at all. The information they seek can range from the effects of outsourcing on individual duties, to the impact of outsourcing on the patient population, to the long-term implications of this sort of decision making on personnel in general. Following is a list of concerns in question format that the communicator will probably need to address:

- What information regarding the outsourcing agreement does a manager need in order to perform his or her job?
- Are there departments that will be affected that have not been involved previously?
- If this information is not disseminated to the managers, will there be any gaps in performance levels?
- How active is the management staff in the surrounding community?
- Do the majority of employees believe they will be working at the facility until retirement?
- When employees hear about this outsourcing agreement, how will their perceptions change?
- What will be the reaction of the community when it learns of the outsourcing agreement? Will it be positive, negative, or indifferent?
- What kind of information could be disseminated to any groups in order to shift public opinion? Which groups should be targeted?

The information needed by each group—management, employees, and community—will vary according to the group's focus. For instance, managers will need to understand the management responsibilities that will fall to the outsourcing firm, while employees of other departments will want to know whether outsourcing is planned for their departments. Supplying such information will decrease the rumors that will invariably arise. More important, there will be less confusion in affected areas, allowing both internal staff and the outsourcing firm to perform to the best of their ability.

COMMUNICATION WITH MANAGEMENT

The first layer of communication must be directed to the management of the organization. This group has many potential roles that can cement the success of the outsourcing agreement. These roles can be categorized as internal and external.

Internal Roles of the Management Staff

The internal roles of the management staff are focused on performing the responsibilities of their positions. They require a certain amount of information about other departments to direct their own areas. Therefore, much of the information that department managers need pertains to how the outsourcing contract will affect them and what role they may play. For instance, if clinical engineering is being outsourced, a number of managers will need to understand how systems may be changed and how their staff will get items repaired. In addition, they will want to understand how responsibilities will dovetail with operations of the rest of the facility. Will the outsourcing firm offer technical expertise on acquisition of new equipment? Will they track warranties?

It is important to remember that many of the management staff may have had no prior exposure to the outsourcing discussion or agreement, and this may cause dissension if they do not feel included. Communication lines must be open in order to establish an atmosphere of cooperation conducive to productivity within their ranks.

External Roles of the Management Staff

Management staff also has ties to the external world through associations, professional groups, and community organizations. In these settings, they are bound to be asked about or hear discussion regarding outsourcing agreements. If they are armed with relevant and accurate information, they can help eliminate negative publicity and contribute to the success of the project. To meet this challenge, managers must be armed with information about the who, why, when, how, and what of the outsourcing contract. They should be conversant with the facts to present the agreement in the best possible light.

COMMUNICATION WITH EMPLOYEES

One purpose of communicating to managers is to use them in public relations roles and thus extend the influence of the administration into the community. When dealing with employees, this is a secondary consideration. The primary consideration is to lessen the anxiety and concerns that may arise as a result of the outsourcing agreement.

Employee Expectations

Many health care organizations have long-time employees who plan to remain with the facility until retirement. As has been seen in other industries, the cradle-to-grave employment philosophy of previous generations is changing, and individuals may work for many different organizations over the course of their working years. However, this trend has not been as prevalent in the health care industry as it has in other industries; therefore, employees must be given assistance to come to terms with this change in the marketplace and its impact on their futures.

Focus of Communication

The focus of communication with the staff should be to provide accurate details of why the outsourcing strategy has been chosen. Some organizations start the information campaign by painting a realistic picture of the financial status of the organization and follow it up by listing the alternate actions that were considered and why they were deemed unworkable. Then the outsourcing contract is discussed: what it means to the institution, how it will be implemented, and what it means to each employee. It is important that this discussion include an overview of the strategic factors that led to the decision to outsource as well as whether outsourcing may be considered for other areas.

COMMUNICATION WITH THE COMMUNITY

The community is potentially the most important group to be considered. These are the individuals who will use health services. Ensuring that they have a positive attitude toward the facility will afford continued growth despite increasing competition. If all other factors are equal between two health care organizations, negative publicity about one may cause patients to choose the other for their health care.

First, the health care organization must determine what the community needs to know. In essence, the users of a health service want assurance that the service levels they are accustomed to will not change, that the local facility they are familiar with will be there, and that outsourcing is not a first step toward closure.

Second, after defining the message it wants to deliver to the community, the health care organization must determine the right media for reaching residents of the service area. For example, radio and television may allow for the widest coverage, but may not be appropriate to reach the target audience. Instead, local newspapers may afford the best link to the inhabitants of the community. In addition, organizational and staff membership in local chambers of commerce and community groups may offer easy access to those people the organization must reach.

COMMUNICATION IN THE HEALTH CARE SYSTEM OF THE FUTURE

Outsourcing results in the creation of an organizational structure that is a dramatic departure from that of the institution that owned, managed, and controlled all of its resources and assets. The health care system of the future will be a network of compartmentalized services unified by a relationship to a central group of managers and professionals who set direction for the organization and coordinate operation of autonomous services.

This central hub will connect the following:

- Decentralized operating units employing full-time in-house staff
- Vendors providing non-core services that make it possible for the health care organization to focus internal efforts on its core competencies
- Strategic vendors providing expertise and services that make it possible for the health care management team to engage in market maneuvers that provide a competitive advantage
- Vendors providing specialized services on an as-needed basis

CONCLUSION

By approaching communication in an organized manner and targeting managers, employees, and the community, a health care organization can help itself and its outsourcing partner by minimizing the negative publicity that can accompany the outsourcing agreement and by tempering employee reactions. An organization that approaches communication in an honest and open manner can turn disconcerting situations into opportunities.

11

Alternatives to Outsourcing

Health care continues to evolve in response to the changing environment, and as it does, the application of outsourcing continues to change as well. While health care executives are adapting outsourcing contracts to meet their needs, they are looking at internal operations in a new light, hoping to capitalize on areas of expertise that may already exist.

This chapter examines three alternatives to outsourcing: cosourcing, insourcing, and returning an outsourced activity to in-house control.

COSOURCING

The term _cosourcing_ has at least two definitions within the health care community: the hiring of an outside firm to manage all outsourcing contracts, and the awarding of responsibility for one activity to two or more vendors.

Outside Management of Outsourcing Contracts

As discussed in chapter 9, hiring an outside consultant to manage outsourcing contracts makes sense in that it lessens the need for administrators to spend large amounts of their time overseeing outsourcing agreements and allows them instead to focus on strategic issues within the organization.

Because one vendor is made responsible for ensuring that each service provider performs to the level required in its contract, all communication between the health care organization and its various vendors is handled by the oversight firm. This approach can be extremely beneficial, especially when an organization has a significant number of outsourcing providers.

The downside is the addition of another layer of management. This can slow communication—already potentially an area of concern. Another issue may be a feeling of losing control by some administrators. While they have accepted the need to outsource a function, they may be reluctant to outsource the management of the function as well. The way to overcome this is to ensure open lines of communication between the oversight firm and internal administrators.

One Activity Awarded to Multiple Vendors

When one activity is awarded to two or more vendors, typically each vendor brings expertise to the table that the other vendor does not possess. For example, in the area of radiology equipment, manufacturers began to offer asset management to their customers at about the same time that other firms began to offer management service for the care of movable medical equipment. Although each activity is a form of asset management, neither firm would have all of the skills needed to provide adequate service. Radiology equipment depends significantly on uptime; therefore, manufacturers would primarily be responsible for the operational aspect of the equipment. However, another aspect of asset management is having movable medical equipment in the right place at the right time. Moving the equipment would require a different vendor. The solution for many facilities is to contract with two firms, one for radiology and the other for movable medical equipment.

Other examples of two-vendor possibilities include:

- Patient and visitor food service
- Accounts payable and accounts receivable
- Internal and external distribution (for example, campus mail service and supply delivery to an entire integrated health care system)

While these double functions are similar, in each case they could be divided and given to two different vendors.

INSOURCING

Insourcing is the awarding of an outsourcing contract to an internal department, though not necessarily to the department that would typically be responsible for the activity. Choosing an internal department over an external vendor can be a solid business decision. Particular activities may be a key component of a department without being the task for which it is most notable. However, when a competency within the department equals or exceeds that of outside sources, the best use of resources would dictate that the activity be assigned to the in-house experts. In some cases, volume that can be transferred from one department to another may eliminate excess capacity while improving the quality of service being provided. Internal departments should be invited to "bid" on outsourcing contracts for the performance of non-core activities at the same time as outside vendors.

Activities that may be considered for insourcing include transcription of surgical reports by the transcription staff in radiology, medical office building cleaning by the housekeeping department, and radiology file management by the medical records department.

An example of an insourcing situation is that of a medical records department of a 250-bed, rural community hospital. The department had received a number of complaints from physicians about the turnaround time on dictation, especially for patient discharge summaries and operative records. The director of the department decided to check with colleagues in other hospitals to determine how they handled this problem. They all explained that they outsourced transcription activity, finding it to be timely and cost-effective.

The director of medical records discussed the issue with the hospital administrator, and they decided that all transcription services in the hospital should be analyzed with an eye toward outsourcing. Areas providing transcription services included medical records, radiology, pathology, business health, and physical therapy. The administrator presented the project to her peers in these departments and requested information with which to compare the various transcription services. To benchmark internal performance, the director of medical records obtained a quote for provision of transcription services from a vendor recommended by her colleagues.

Based on the information obtained from the internal review of all transcription services, it was determined that one internal department—radiology—functioned at a higher level than that offered by the outside vendor. This indicated that the radiology department had the expertise required to improve the quality of work internally in a cost-effective manner.

The administrator made the following recommendations:

- Treat the provision of transcription as an outsourced service in all areas except radiology. This will require development of performance standards to conduct ongoing performance tests.
- Centralize transcription services under the radiology department.
- Treat provisions of transcription services as a revenue-generating contract within radiology. Assign responsibility for profit and loss to the department administrator.
- Monitor performance as if the contract were assigned to an outside vendor.

RETURNING AN OUTSOURCED ACTIVITY TO IN-HOUSE CONTROL

The latest development in outsourcing is the return of an outsourced department to in-house control and operation. Organizations report that in some instances they have found it to be more cost-effective to perform an activity internally than to contract it to an outsider. Other facilities bring a function in-house when what was once considered a peripheral activity assumes greater importance because of market changes.

To Reduce Cost

The primary reason for outsourcing is not to reduce cost, although this is usually a secondary benefit. Rather, outsourcing is a strategy that allows the health care organization to capitalize on the expertise of other firms to perform a task so that the organization can focus its internal efforts on its core competencies. However, simply regaining internal control over an activity does little to meet this objective. Therefore, returning an activity to in-house control is typically done to reduce cost.

When the cost of an outsourced activity exceeds that of projected internal cost, the health care organization should determine why the cost for outside performance rose at a faster rate than internal costs. If the activity was less expensive using external providers when the contract was signed, it should never exceed internal costs. However, organizations often discover that the original contract was not as cost-effective as previously believed. For example, some hospitals discovered this problem when they opted to outsource information services. When the contracts were signed originally, cost projections seemed appropriate; however, as time went by and the cost of hardware and software dropped significantly, costs soared compared with those that would be expected if the services were returned to in-house control. For these organizations, bringing the activity in-house would be cost-effective.

To Respond to Market Changes

When an organization chooses a new path, some outsourced activities may become of greater interest as core competencies are redefined. Such changes often occur in clinical areas. For example, one facility decided to outsource its physical therapy department. At the time, there were no in-house programs that demanded this expertise, nor was physical therapy deemed to be a core competency. Some years later, the organization changed its course as a result of a competitive market analysis. There was an opportunity to establish an occupational health program, and physical therapy was deemed to be a critical element of the program.

This institution had two choices in responding to the increased importance of physical therapy. The first was to bring the activity back in-house and develop the expertise needed to provide effective therapy. The alternative was to approach the physical therapy outsourcing vendor and discuss the opportunity to expand the vendor's responsibilities. Working together might provide both organizations with financial rewards.

More important, such an approach does not require capital investments by the hospital and allows the managers to concentrate on the task of establishing an effective occupational health program rather than focusing on regaining control of the physical therapy department.

Whether to reduce cost or to respond to market changes, deciding to return an outsourced activity to in-house control involves considering questions such as:

- Will current management structure allow for optimal performance?
- What other projects is the administrator who will manage this activity responsible for?
- What other activities might be overlooked or receive less attention if this activity is moved in-house?
- What resources will be required to successfully perform this activity in-house?
- Has the importance of this activity changed in relation to the organization's strategic plan?

The last question demands scrutiny. Over time, priorities change, and the importance of any outsourced activity should be reconsidered when they do. However, in most instances, activities that are outsourced are of less importance to the primary focus of the institution unless the organization chooses a significantly new direction.

CONCLUSION

Outsourcing introduces flexibility into an organization and opens up the potential of cosourcing, insourcing, or redirecting the activity to in-house staff. Properly researched and implemented, it can be the keystone of the hospital organization's success, illuminating its strengths and weaknesses, and providing a focus on core competencies that will improve productivity and ensure patient satisfaction.

Index